Mabel Cavaiani, R.D.
Muriel Urbashich, R.D.

Simplified Quantity Recipes

Nursing/Convalescent Homes and Hospitals

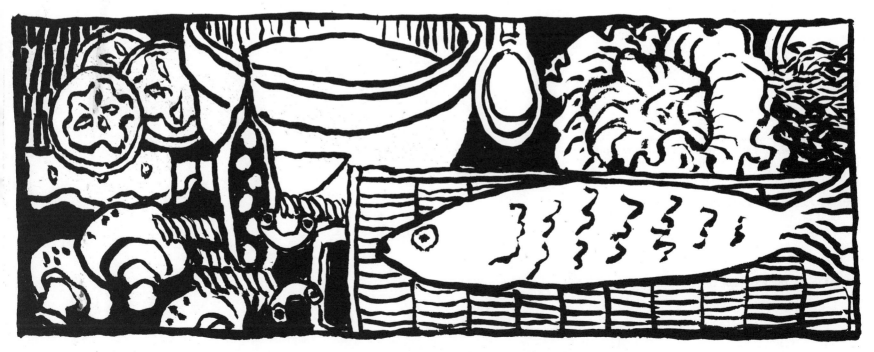

Published by the National Restaurant Association

Published by
National Restaurant Association
311 First St., N.W.
Washington, DC 20001

ISBN 0-914528-05-X

Printed in the United States of America

Table of Contents

Foreword

Simplified Quantity Recipes provides for the foodservice industry a concise, usable, quantity recipe book for the operators who are challenged by cost containment and who oftentimes find themselves with eager but not professionally trained employees.

This book is tangible evidence of response to the needs in the industry for a simplified, standard, quantity recipe book complete with information on diabetic exchanges and other nutritional information.

The authors Mabel Cavaiani and Muriel Urbashich are recognized authorities in the field of nursing/convalescent homes and hospitals, and have extended to the industry and to you, the reader, an invaluable service.

WILLIAM P. FISHER
Executive Vice President
National Restaurant Association

Introduction and Acknowledgements

This book was written in response to the need for simplified, standardized recipes suitable for nursing/convalescent homes and hospitals. Dietary information is included for the convenience of food service supervisors who do not have a dietitian available at all times. An explanation of the various diets and other dietary information is included in chapter one "Dietary Information."

Recipes in this second edition have been changed, when necessary, to reflect an emphasis on recipes with lower calories, sugar and saturated fat. Fiber has been increased whenever possible and new recipes have been included for cakes, cookies and hot breads to provide a good source of fiber acceptable to the residents in the home or hospital.

Recipes in this book are also suitable for cafeterias, schools, restaurants and others wanting recipes for wholesome, nutritious, attractive and economical food. Recipes have been simplified as much as possible for the housewife turned cook and other employees without formal education in food preparation. Basic, simple equipment has been used and terms and measures have been spelled out. Yields reflect generally accepted portions for nursing/convalescent homes and can be increased or decreased as necessary using the directions in the information chapter. An extra column has been provided beside the Weights and Measures column to record the adjusted amounts. All measures and portions are level and it should be emphasized that correct yields, particularly for meats, cannot be expected unless the correct temperatures and equipment are used.

The authors would like to give special thanks for help and encouragement in the preparation of this book and its first revision to the following persons and organizations.

Donna Beckstrom, Vice President of Golden West Medical Nutrition Center, Newport Beach, California.

Dorothy Berzy, R.D., Nutrition Care Dietitian and **Diane R. Billmeyer, R.D.,** Chief Clinical Dietitian, South Chicago Community Hospital, Chicago, Illinois.

Mary Jane Chivers, R.D., former Nutrition Instructor and Administrative Assistant, Christ Hospital, Oak Lawn, Illinois.

Frances Lee, M.S., R.D., Dietary Consultant, Kerens, Texas.

Frances Nielsen, former Food Service Supervisor, Bridgeview, Illinois.

Mary Agnes Jones, R.D., Chief Administrative Dietitian, Holy Cross Hospital, Chicago, Illinois.

Betty Jane Walter, R.D., Dietary Consultant, Jackson, Michigan.

Mary Klicka, M.S., R.D, Chief, **Patricia Prell, M.S., R.D.** and **Jessie McNutt, R.D.,** The Ration Design and Evaluation Branch, U.S. Army, Natick Research and Development Center, Natick, Mass.

The Administrator, Food Service Supervisor and Dietary Staff of The Lutheran Home and Gernand Retirement Center, Strawberry Point, Iowa.

The Food Service Supervisor and Dietary Staff of Healthcare Manor, New Hampton, Iowa.

Nutrient Data Research Branch, Human Nutrition Information Service, U.S. Department of Agriculture.

Armed Forces Recipe Service Committee.

U.S. Department of Agriculture, School Lunch Program.

U.S. Department of Commerce, National Marine Fisheries Institute.

National Livestock and Meat Board.

American Dry Milk Institute.

National Turkey Federation.

Chapter 1
Dietary Information

Optimum nutrition in the home, hospital or nursing/convalescent home is an essential. It is becoming more apparent that adequate nutrition is vital to good health and the prevention of disease throughout our lives.

Food also represents a great deal more such as love, security, happiness, sociability, and is an integral part of many religious and ethnic groups.

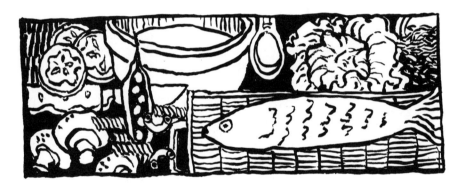

Dietary Information

It is particularly important that quality be stressed in the preparation of food to be served in nursing/convalescent homes and hospitals where so many of the familiar, reassuring surroundings are absent and the guests or patients are totally dependent on nutritionally adequate meals. The diet should be adequate in all nutrients according to the National Research Council's recommended daily dietary allowances and the government's recommended guidelines which follow:

1. Eat a variety of foods.
2. Maintain desirable weight.
3. Avoid too much fat, saturated fat, and cholesterol.
4. Eat foods with adequate starch and fiber.
5. Avoid too much sugar.
6. Avoid too much sodium.
7. If you drink alcoholic beverages, do so in moderation.

It is vital to maintain the patient or resident at a sound nutritional state through adequate caloric and protein intake.

Nutrition information is furnished at the bottom of recipes in this book. It is for the basic recipe only and not for any variations. The dietary information in each recipe is based on information taken from the Manual of Clinical Dietetics, researched and approved by the South Suburban Dietetic Association and Chicago Dietetic Association of Cook and Will Counties.

Nutritive information in this book is based upon information in the following U.S. government publications, except as noted otherwise.

NUTRITIVE VALUE OF AMERICAN FOODS IN COMMON UNITS, AGRICULTURAL HANDBOOK 456, U.S. Department of Agriculture, Washington, D.C., Superintendent of Documents, U.S. Government Printing Office, 1975.

NUTRITIVE VALUE OF FOODS, HOME AND GARDEN BULLETIN 72, U.S. Department of Agriculture, Washington, D.C., Superintendent of Documents, U.S. Government Printing Office.

COMPOSITION OF FOODS, RAW, PROCESSED AND PREPARED, AGRICULTURE HANDBOOK NO. 8, U.S. Department of Agriculture, Washington, D.C., Superintendent of Documents, U.S. Government Printing Office, 1963, and as many of the current revisions as are available at this time.

You will note strict dietary regimens are not followed for nursing/convalescent homes. It is suggested that if a specific food causes distress for a patient then that food should be eliminated from his or her diet. In hospitals you will encounter illnesses that require more strict dietary modification. In this case the dietitian can make those adjustments in the recipes or on the daily menus.

Nutrition assessments are done to evaluate the needs of all patients or guests.

COST-EFFECTIVE QUALITY FOOD SERVICE

There is no food service department that cannot reduce costs, and analyzing the department is the first step toward cost containment. Many nursing homes and hospitals are concerned about the drop in census. Many of them are trying to increase revenue to compensate for the census reduction in such ways as paid catering, special take-home meals, selling meat platters for parties, producing party cakes, and charging for community services, such as wellness programs and classes for people on special diets.

In addition to revenue-producing ideas, it is possible to help achieve cost containment by using good management techniques such as the following:

A. Realistic budgeting.
B. Flexible and creative scheduling.
C. Training programs and training employees to be capable of handling more than one job.
D. Analyzing the cost of china versus disposable and checking the cost of china now being used.
E. Using a shorter menu cycle with a nonselective menu.
F. Planning menus based on the goals of your organization, whether those goals are to save money, serve the best meals available, cater to ethnic groups or provide meals which are economical as well as attractive and healthy.
G. Controlling cost by use of standard recipes.
H. Close inventory control to prevent waste.
I. Purchasing and utilizing specifications and group purchasing.
J. Accurate receiving and disbursements.
K. Analyzing production sheets detailing activities of the day.
L. Ingredient and portion control.
M. Checking nourishment costs and setting up realistic lists of nourishments.

HIGH-FIBER DIET

In the last 15 years there seems to be an increasing awareness of the value of fiber in the diet. High-fiber diets, it is thought, play a role in the prevention of cardiovascular disease, diabetes, obesity and intestinal disease.

A considerable amount of research is being done in this area. A high-fiber diet at this time is being used in relieving the symptoms of diverticular disease, atonic constipation and treatment of irritable bowel syndrome.

SODIUM-CONTROLLED DIETS

Sodium-controlled diets are generally utilized to prevent excessive sodium retention which in turn may result in fluid retention caused by cardiovascular, renal or hepatic disease. There are five levels of sodium modification in the Manual of Clinical Dietetics.

This book is directed primarily at nursing/convalescent homes. The average patient in a nursing home in the United States is 81 years old. For these persons strict therapeutic diet regimens have not proven to be of significant value. Therefore, in this book we will use modification #1 in the Manual of Clinical Dietetics which is titled "No Added Salt." It contains approximately 4 gm. sodium. All foods on the general diet are used but salt is not given at the table. It is suggested foods highly salted or preserved in salt be limited or eliminated. It is also recommended soups be made from beef bones or chicken necks and backs if possible, the product being far superior for all diets and lower in sodium content than stock made from regular commercial bases.

BLAND DIET

Purpose: The diet for chronic peptic ulcer is designated to provide a nutritionally adequate diet by restricting or avoiding foods that may cause gastric irritation and excessive gastric acid secretion.
Modification: The following modifications are made:

1. Three regular meals are recommended.
2. Avoidance of between-meal and especially bedtime snacks, as they interfere with antacid therapy.
3. Neutralization of the effect of restricted foods, which increase gastric acid secretion, by ingesting them at or near mealtimes.
4. There is little rationale for completely eliminating any foods from the diet unless a particular food causes an individual repeated discomfort. Caffeine-containing beverages (coffee, tea, and cola drinks) and decaffeinated coffee cause increased gastric acid production but may be taken in moderation at or near mealtime, if tolerated.
5. Excessive alcohol intake should be avoided because of the damaging effect it has on the gastric mucosal lining. Contrary to past belief, alcohol has not been shown to increase gastric acid secretion in humans. Until further research shows that alcohol has damaging, neutral, or even beneficial effects in peptic ulcers, it should be eliminated from the diet or taken in moderation at or near mealtimes, if tolerated.
6. Black, white or red pepper, chili powder, chocolate, peppers, cloves, nutmeg and nicotine may cause distress and may have to be avoided.

This entire page thru section 5 has been taken from the Manual of Clinical Dietetics, Section 4, Gastrointestinal Diets, pages 55 & 56.

LOWFAT DIET 40-45 gms.

The lowfat diet is utilized to achieve a level of 40-45 gms. of fat per day in the individual's meal pattern. The diet may be used for diseases of the liver, gallbladder, pancreas and also weight reduction. The amount of fat in the recipes in this book has been restricted so the recipes might be used as much as possible for patients on a lowfat regimen.

All visible fat should be removed from meat and the skin should be removed from poultry.

This 40-45 gms. lowfat diet would naturally eliminate foods with a high fat content. Foods also that cause gaseous distention may have to be omitted.

It must be noted these recipes are a segment only of the entire day's intake of 40-45 gms. of fat.

LOW CHOLESTEROL DIET

This diet is utilized to reduce serum lipid levels. It follows a general diet with specific adjustments.

The following guidelines should be followed:

Foods excluded —

Whole milk, products made with whole milk, 2% and lowfat milk, chocolate milk, evaporated and condensed milk, and cream.

Egg breads, butter rolls, popovers, snack crackers and other snack foods, commercial granola cereals, biscuits, muffins, doughnuts, French toast, sweet rolls, and any others made with egg yolks, butter, coconut oil, whole milk or cream.

Fried potatoes, potato chips, egg or chow mein noodles, fried rice (except with allowed oils).

Duck, goose, fatty meats, bacon, corned beef, spareribs, luncheon meats, frankfurters and other sausage, canned meats, liver and other organ meats, shrimp, caviar, sardines, cream cheese, pre-basted or pre-stuffed poultry, TV dinners, convenience foods and commercially prepared foods unless labeled as containing polyunsaturated fat.

Butter, cream, sour cream, whipping cream, lard, salt pork, bacon fat and all products containing animal fat, coconut oil, and any products containing them except those included.

Soups made with whole milk or cream.

Ice cream and ice milk, commercial pie, cakes, cookies and mixes.

Any candy or dessert made with chocolate, whole milk, cream or coconut.

Beverages containing whole milk, cream or chocolate.

Gravies and sauce unless made with allowed oils and/or skim milk.

Chocolate, coconut, cashews, macadamia nuts, pork rinds.

The entire previous section was taken from the Manual of Clinical Dietetics, pages 189, 190 & 191.

LACTOSE-RESTRICTED DIET

The lactose-restricted diet is designated to provide foods that contain a minimal amount of lactose.

It is used for patients who do not tolerate lactose because of a deficiency of lactase. The severity of symptoms depends on the quantity of lactose consumed and the extent of lactase deficiency.

The diet is a general diet with the elimination of milk and milk products (lactose-containing foods). Read labels. Avoid any foods containing lactose, milk, or milk solids. Lactate, lactalbumin, lactylate, and calcium compounds are salts of lactic acid and do not contain lactose. Foods processed with small amounts of milk, milk solids, or lactose may be used with discretion if tolerated.

Soybean milks and other lactose-free supplements can be utilized.

Buttermilk and yogurt may be tolerated by some individuals.

This section has been taken from the Manual of Clinical Dietetics, pages 71 & 72.

MECHANICAL SOFT DIET

The mechanical soft diet is utilized for those individuals who are unable to chew their food sufficiently. The recipes in this book have been analyzed in regard to their usage on the mechanical soft diet. Where applicable it is suggested they be used. The patient should be visited by a dietitian to determine his or her ability to handle a specific food.

GERIATRIC DIET

The geriatric diet follows the general diet and is used for persons not requiring specific dietary modifications. Because of a decrease in basal metabolic rate, lean body mass and physical activity, it is recommended calorie content be reduced as well as fat content. Avoidance of fried foods is recommended. Foods should be colorful, well-seasoned and attractively served. It is wise to emphasize intake of raw and cooked fruits and vegetables, whole grain cereals and breads and sufficient fluids.

SOFT DIET

This diet is used for patients who cannot tolerate a general diet. Fried foods, raw fruits and vegetables, coarse breads and cereals and highly seasoned foods may cause distress and so are eliminated on the soft diet.

LIBERAL DIABETIC DIET

1. Eliminate sugar and concentrated sweets.
2. Serve regular meals and snacks.
3. Decrease total fat intake.
4. Maintain ideal body weight.

This is basically a general diet without concentrated sweets, high fat or fried foods.

DIABETIC DIET

Recipes in this book have been analyzed for milk, vegetable, fruit, bread, meat and fat exchanges.

When it is possible to use the recipe for diabetic patients, the pertinent exchanges are listed. If the recipes are considered too high in some exchanges to be used for diabetic diets, no exchanges are listed. When the quantities of a particular food group are negligible they are not mentioned in the exchanges listed at the end of the recipe.

The "Exchange Lists for Meal Planning" are on the next page.

Starch / Bread List

Each item in this list contains approximately 15 grams of carbohydrate, 3 grams of protein, a trace of fat and 80 calories.

Whole grain products average about 2 grams of fiber per serving. Some foods are higher in fiber. Those foods that contain 3 or more grams of fiber per serving are identified with the fiber symbol *.

You can choose your starch exchanges from any of the items on this list. If you want to eat a starch food that is not on this list, the general rule is that:

½ cup of cereal, grain or pasta is one serving

1 ounce of a bread product is one serving.

Your dietitian can help you be more exact.

Cereals / Grains / Pasta:

Bran cereals*, concentrated	⅓ cup
Bran cereals*, flaked (such as Bran Buds_R, All Bran_R)	½ cup
Bulgur (cooked)	½ cup
Cooked cereals	½ cup
Cornmeal (dry)	2½ Tbsp.
Grapenuts	3 Tbsp.
Grits (cooked)	½ cup
Other ready-to-eat unsweetened cereals	¾ cup
Pasta (cooked)	½ cup
Puffed cereal	1½ cup
Rice, white or brown (cooked)	⅓ cup
Shredded wheat	½ cup
Wheat germ*	3 Tbsp.

Dried Beans, Peas / Lentils:

Beans* and peas* (cooked) such as kidney, white, split, blackeye	⅓ cup
Lentils* (cooked)	⅓ cup
Baked beans*	¼ cup

Starchy Vegetables:

Corn*	½ cup
Corn on cob*, 6″ long	1
Lima beans*	½ cup
Peas, green* (canned or frozen)	½ cup
Plantain*	½ cup
Potato, baked	1 small (3 oz.)
Potato, mashed	½ cup
Squash, winter* (acorn, butternut)	¾ cup
Yam, sweet potato, plain	⅓ cup

Bread:

Bagel	½ (1 oz.)
Bread sticks, crisp, 4″ long × ½″	2 (⅔ oz.)
Croutons, low fat	1 cup
English muffin	½
Frankfurter or hamburger bun	½ (1 oz.)
Pita, 6″ across	½
Plain roll, small	1 (1 oz.)
Raisin, unfrosted	1 slice (1 oz.)
Rye*, pumpernickel*	1 slice (1 oz.)
Tortilla, 6″ across	1
White (including French, Italian)	1 slice (1 oz.)
Whole wheat	1 slice (1 oz.)

Crackers / Snacks:

Animal crackers	8
Graham crackers, 2½″ square	3
Matzoth	¾ oz.
Melba toast	5 slices
Oyster crackers	24
Popcorn (popped, no fat added)	3 cups
Preetzels	¾ oz.
Rye crisp, 2″ × 3-½″	4
Saltine-type crackers	6
Whole wheat crackers, no fat added (crisp breads, such as Finn_R, Kavli_R, Wasa_R)	2-4 slices (¾ oz.)

Starch Foods Prepared With Fat:
(Count as 1 starch/bread serving, plus 1 fat serving.)

Biscuit, 2½″ across	1
Chow mein noodles	½ cup
Corn bread, 2″ cube	1 (2 oz.)

Cracker, round butter type	6
French fried potatoes, 2″ to 3-1/2″ long	10 (1½ oz.)
Muffin, plain, small	1
Pancake, 4″ across	2
Stuffing, bread (prepared)	¼ cup
Taco shell, 6″ across	2
Waffle, 4½″ square	1
Whole wheat crackers, fat added (such as Triscuits_R)	4-6 (1 oz.)

*3 grams or more of fiber per serving.

Meat List

Each serving of meat and substitutes on this list contains about 7 grams of protein. The amount of fat and number of calories varies, depending on what kind of meat or substitute you choose. The list is divided into three parts based on the amount of fat and calories: lean meat, medium-fat meat and high-fat meat. One ounce (one meat exchange) of each of these includes:

	Carbohydrate (grams)	Protein (grams)	Fat (grams)	Calories
Lean	0	7	3	55
Medium-Fat	0	7	5	75
High-Fat	0	7	8	100

You are encouraged to use more lean and medium-fat meat, poultry and fish in your meal plan. This will help decrease your fat intake, which may help decrease your risk for heart diesase. The items from the high-fat group are high in saturated fat, cholesterol and calories. You should limit your choices from the high-fat group to 3 times per week. Meat and substitutes do not contribute any fiber to your meal plan.

Tips:

1. Bake, roast, broil, grill or boil these foods rather than frying them with added fat.
2. Use a nonstick pan spray or a nonstick pan to brown or fry these foods.
3. Trim off visible fat before and after cooking.
4. Do not add flour, bread crumbs, coating mixes or fat to these foods when preparing them.
5. Weigh meat after removing bones and fat, and after cooking. Three ounces of cooked meat is about equal to 4 ounces of raw meat. Some examples of meat portions are:

2 ounces meat (2 meat exchanges) — 1 small chicken leg or thigh
½ cup cottage cheese or tuna

3 ounces meat (3 meat exchanges — 1 medium pork chop
1 small hamburger
½ of a whole chicken breast
1 unbreaded fish fillet
cooked meat, about the size of a deck of cards

6. Restaurants usually serve prime cuts of meat, which are high in fat and calories.

Lean Meat and Substitutes
(One exchange is equal to any one of the following items.)

Beef:	USDA Good or Choice grades of lean beef, such as round, sirloin and flank steak; tenderloin; and chipped beef**.	1 oz.
Pork:	Lean pork, such as fresh ham; canned, cured or boiled ham;** Canadian bacon**, tenderloin.	1 oz.
Veal:	All cuts are lean except for veal cutlets (ground or cubed). Examples of lean veal are chops and roasts.	1 oz.
Poultry:	Chicken, turkey, Cornish hen (without skin)	1 oz.
Fish:	All fresh and frozen fish	1 oz.
	Crab, lobster, scallops, shrimp, clams (fresh or canned in water**)	2 oz.
	Oysters	6 medium
	Tuna** (canned in water)	¼ cup
	Salmon** (canned)	¼ cup
	Herring (uncreamed or smoked)	1 oz.
	Sardines (canned)	2 medium
Wild Game:	Venison, rabbit, squirrel	1 oz.
	Pheasant, duck, goose (without skin)	1 oz.

Cheese:	Any cottage cheese	¼ cup
	Grated parmesan	2 Tbsp.
	Diet cheeses** with less than 55 calories per ounce	1 oz.
Other:	95% fat-free luncheon meat**	1 oz.
	Egg whites	3 whites
	Egg substitutes with less than 55 calories per ¼ cup	¼ cup

Medium-Fat Meat and Substitutes
(One exchange is equal to any one of the following items.)

Beef:	Most beef products fall into this category. Examples are: all ground beef, roast (rib, chuck, rump), steak (cubed, Porterhouse, T-Bone) and meatloaf.	1 oz.
Pork:	Most pork products fall into this category. Examples are: chops, loin roast, Boston butt, cutlets.	1 oz.
Lamb:	Most lamb products fall into this category. Examples are: chops, leg and roast.	1 oz.
Veal:	Cutlet (ground or cubed, unbreaded)	1 oz.
Poultry:	Chicken (with skin), domestic duck or goose (well-drained of fat), ground turkey	1 oz.
Fish:	Tuna** (canned in oil and drained)	¼ cup
	Salmon** (canned)	¼ cup
Cheese:	Skim or part-skim milk cheeses, such as:	
	Ricotta	¼ cup
	Mozzarella	1 oz.
	Diet cheeses** with 56–80 calories per ounce	1 oz.
Other:	86% fat-free luncheon meat**	1 oz.
	Egg (high in cholesterol, limit to 3 per week)	1
	Egg substitutes with 56–80 calories per ¼ cup	¼ cup
	Tofu (2-½″ × 2-¾″ × 1″)	4 oz.
	Liver, heart, kidney, sweetbreads (high in cholesterol)	1 oz.

High-Fat Meat and Substitutes
Remember, these items are high in saturated fat, cholesterol, and calories and should be used only 3 times per week. (One exchange is equal to any one of the following items.)

Beef:	Most USDA Prime cuts of beef, such as ribs, corned beef.**	1 oz.
Pork:	Spareribs, ground pork, pork sausage** (patty or link)	1 oz.
Lamb:	Patties (ground lamb)	1 oz.
Fish:	Any fried fish product	1 oz.
Cheese:	All regular cheeses,** such as American, Blue, Cheddar, Monterey, Swiss	1 oz.
Other:	Luncheon meat,** such as bologna, salami, pimento loaf	1 oz.
	Sausage**, such as Polish, Italian, Knockwurst, smoked	1 oz.
	Bratwurst**	1 oz.
	Frankfurter** (turkey or chicken)	1 frank (10/lb.)
	Peanut butter (contains unsaturated fat)	1 Tbsp.

Count as one high-fat meat plus one fat exchange:

| | Frankfurter** (beef, pork, or combination) | 1 frank (10/lb.) |

**Meats and meat substitutes that have 400 milligrams or more of sodium per exchange are indicated with this symbol.

Vegetable List

Each vegetable serving on this list contains about 5 grams of carbohydrate, 2 grams of protein, and 25 calories. Vegetables contain 2-3 grams of dietary fiber. Vegetables which contain 400 mg or more of sodium per serving are identified with a ** symbol.

Vegetables are a good source of vitamins and minerals. Fresh and frozen vegetables have more vitamins and less added salt. Rinsing canned vegetables will remove much of the salt.

Unless otherwise noted, the serving size for vegetables (one vegetable exchange) is:

½ cup of cooked vegetables or vegetable juice
1 cup of raw vegetables

Artichoke (½ medium)	Eggplant	Rutabaga
Asparagus	Greens (collard, mustard, turnip)	Sauerkraut**
Beans (green, wax, Italian)	Kohlrabi	Spinach, cooked
Bean sprouts	Leeksk	Summer squash (crookneck)
Beets	Mushrooms, cooked	Tomato (one large)
Broccoli	Okra	Tomato/vegetable juice**
Brussels sprouts	Onions	Turnips
Cabbage, cooked	Pea pods	Water chestnuts
Carrots	Peppers (green)	Zucchini, cooked
Cauliflower		

Starchy vegetables such as corn, peas, and potatoes are found on the Starch/Bread List.

For free vegetables, see Free Food List on page 19.

**400 mg or more of sodium per serving

Fruit List

Each item on this list contains about 15 grams of carbohydrate, and 60 calories. Fresh, frozen, and dry fruits have about 2 grams of fiber per serving. Fruits that have 3 or more grams of fiber per serving have a * symbol. Fruit juices contain very little dietary fiber.

The carbohydrate and calorie content for a fruit serving are based on the usual serving of the most commonly eaten fruits. Use fresh fruits or fruits frozen or canned without sugar added. Whole fruit is more filling than fruit juice and may be a better choice for those who are trying to lose weight. Unless otherwise noted, the serving size for one fruit serving is:

> ½ cup of fresh fruit or fruit juice
> ¼ cup of dried fruit

Fresh, frozen, and unsweetened canned fruit:

Apple, raw, 2" across	1 apple
Applesauce (unsweetened)	½ cup
Apricots (medium, raw) or	4 apricots
Apricots (canned)	½ cup, or 4 halves
Banana (9" long)	½ banana
*Blackberries (raw)	¾ cup
*Blueberries (raw)	¾ cup
Cantaloupe (5" across) (cubes)	⅓ melon 1 cup
Cherries (large, raw)	12 cherries
Figs (raw, 2" across)	2 figs
Fruit cocktail (canned)	½ cup
Grapefruit (medium)	½ grapefruit
Grapefruit (segments)	¾ cup
Grapes (small)	15 grapes
Honeydew melon (medium) (cubes)	⅛ melon 1 cup
Kiwi (large)	1 kiwi
Mandarin oranges	¾ cup
Mango (small)	½ mango
Nectarine, (1-½" across)	1 nectarine
Orange (2-½" across)	1 orange
Papaya	1 cup
Peach (2¾" across)	1 peach
Peaches (canned)	½ cup, 2 halves
Pear	½ large, 1 small
Pears (canned)	½ cup or 2 halves
Persimmon (medium, native)	2 persimmons
Pineapple (raw)	¾ cup
Pineapple (canned)	⅓ cup
Plum (raw, 2" across)	2 plums
*Pomegranate	½ pomegranate
*Raspberries (raw)	1 cup
*Strawberries (raw, whole)	1-¼ cup
Tangerine (2-½" across)	2 tangerines
Watermelon (cubes)	1-¼ cup

Dried Fruit:

*Apples	4 rings
*Apricots	7 halves
Dates	2-1/2 medium
*Figs	1-1/2
*Prunes	3 medium
Raisins	2 Tbsp.

Fruit Juice:

Apple juice/cider	1/2 cup
Cranberry juice cocktail	1/3 cup
Grapefruit juice	1/2 cup
Grape juice	1/3 cup
Orange juice	1/2 cup
Pineapple juice	1/2 cup
Prune juice	1/3 cup

* 3 or more grams of fiber per serving

Milk List

Each serving of milk or milk products on this list contains about 12 grams of carbohydrate and 8 grams of protein. The amount of fat in milk is measured in percent of butterfat. The calories vary, depending on what kind of milk you choose. The list is divided into three parts based on the amount of fat and calories: skim/very lowfat milk, lowfat milk, and whole milk. One serving (one milk exchange) of each of these includes:

	Carbohydrate (grams)	Protein (grams)	Fat (grams)	Calories
Skim/Very Lowfat	12	8	trace	90
Lowfat	12	8	5	120
Whole	12	8	8	150

Milk is the body's main source of calcium, the mineral needed for growth and repair of bones. Yogurt is also a good source of calcium. Yogurt and many dry or powdered milk products have different amounts of fat. If you have questions about a particular item, read the label to find out the fat and calorie content.

Milk is good to drink, but it can also be added to cereal, and to other foods. Many tasty dishes such as sugar-free pudding are made with milk (see the Combination Foods list). Add life to plain yogurt by adding one of your fruit servings to it.

Skim and Very Lowfat Milk:

Skim milk	1 cup
1/2% milk	1 cup
1% milk	1 cup
Lowfat buttermilk	1 cup
Evaporated skim milk	1/2 cup
Dry nonfat milk	1/3 cup
Plain nonfat yogurt	8 oz.

Lowfat Milk:

2% milk	1 cup fluid
Plain lowfat yogurt (with added nonfat milk solids)	8 oz.

Whole Milk:

The whole milk group has much more fat per serving than the skim and lowfat groups. Whole milk has more than 3 1/4% butterfat. Try to limit your choices from the whole milk group as much as possible.

Whole milk	1 cup
Evaporated whole milk	1/2 cup
Whole plain yogurt	8 oz.

Fat List

Each serving on the fat list contains about 5 grams of fat and 45 calories.

The foods on the fat list contain mostly fat, although some items may also contain a small amount of protein. All fats are high in calories and should be carefully measured. Everyone should modify their fat intake by eating unsaturated fats instead of saturated fats. The sodium content of these foods varies widely. Check the label for sodium information.

Unsaturated Fats:

Avocado	1/8 medium
Margarine	1 tsp.
+ Margarine, diet	1 Tbsp.
Mayonnaise	1 tsp.
+ Mayonnaise, reduced-calorie	1 Tbsp.
Nuts and Seeds:	
Almonds, dry roasted	6 whole
Cashews, dry roasted	1 Tbsp.
Pecans	2 whole
Peanuts	20 small or 10 large
Walnuts	2 whole
Other nuts	1 Tbsp.
Seeds, pine nuts, sunflower	1 Tbsp.
(without shells)	
Pumpkin seeds	2 tsp.
Oil (corn, cottonseed, safflower, soybean,	1 tsp.
sunflower, olive, peanut)	
+ Olives	10 small or 5 large
Salad dressing, mayonnaise-type	2 tsp.
Salad dressing, mayonnaise-type,	1 Tbsp.
reduced-calorie	
+ Salad dressing (all varieties)	1 Tbsp.
**Salad dressing, reduced-calorie	2 Tbsp.

(Two tablespoons of low-calorie salad dressing is a free food.)

Saturated Fats:

Butter	1 tsp.
+ Bacon	1 slice
Chitterlings	1/2 ounce
Coconut, shredded	2 Tbsp.
Coffee whitener, liquid	2 Tbsp.
Coffee whitener, powder	4 tsp.
Cream (light, coffee, table)	2 Tbsp.
Cream, sour	2 Tbsp.
Cream (heavy, whipping)	1 Tbsp.
Cream cheese	1 Tbsp.
+ Salt pork	1/4 ounce

+ If more than one or two servings are eaten, these foods have 400 mg. or more of sodium.

** 400 mg. or more of sodium per serving.

Combination Foods

Much of the food we eat is mixed together in various combinations. These combination foods do not fit into only one exchange list. It can be quite hard to tell what is in a certain casserole dish or baked food item. This is a list of average values for some typical combination foods. This list will help you fit these foods into your meal plan. Ask your dietitian for information about any other foods you'd like to eat. The *American Diabetes Association/American Dietetic Association Family Cookbooks* and the *American Diabetes Association Holiday Cookbook* have many recipes and further information about many foods, including combination foods. Check your library or local bookstore.

Food	Amount	Exchanges
Casseroles, homemade	1 cup (8 oz.)	2 starch, 2 medium-fat meat, 1 fat
Cheese pizza** thin crust	1/4 of 15 oz. or 1/4 of 10″	2 starch, 1 medium-fat meat, 1 fat
Chili with beans* ** (commercial)	1 cup (8 oz.)	2 starch, 2 medium-fat meat, 2 fat
Chow mein* ** (without noodles or rice)	2 cups (16 oz.)	1 starch, 2 vegetable, 2 lean meat
Macaroni and cheese**	1 cup (8 oz.)	2 starch, 1 medium-fat meat, 2 fat
Soup:		
Bean* **	1 cup (8 oz.)	1 starch, I vegetable, 1 lean meat
Chunky, all varieties**	10-3/4 oz. can	1 starch, 1 vegetable, 1 medium-fat meat
Cream** (made with water)	1 cup (8 oz.)	1 starch, 1 fat
Vegetable** or broth**	1 cup (8 oz.)	1 starch

Spaghetti and meatballs** (canned)	1 cup (8 oz.)	2 starch, 1 medium-fat meat, 1 fat
Sugar-free pudding (made with skim milk)	½ cup	1 starch

If beans are used as a meat substitute:
Dried beans,* peas,* lentils* 1 cup (cooked) 2 starch, 1 lean meat

*   3 grams or more of fiber per serving
** 400 mg or more of sodium per serving

Foods For Occasional Use

Moderate amounts of some foods can be used in your meal plan, in spite of their sugar or fat content, as long as you can maintain blood-glucose control. The following list includes average exchange values for some of these foods. Because they are concentrated sources of carbohydrate, you will notice that the portion sizes are very small. Check with your dietitian for advice on how often and when you can eat them.

Food	Amount	Exchanges
Angel food cake	1/12 cake	2 starch
Cake, no icing	1/12 cake, or a 3″ square	2 starch, 2 fat
Cookies	2 small (1-3/4″ across)	1 starch, 1 fat
Frozen fruit yogurt	1/3 cup	1 starch
Gingersnaps	3	1 starch
Granola	¼ cup	1 starch, 1 fat
Granola bars	1 small	1 starch, 1 fat
Ice cream, any flavor	½ cup	1 starch, 2 fat
Ice milk, any flavor	½ cup	1 starch, 1 fat
Sherbet, any flavor	¼ cup	1 starch
Snack chips,** all varieties	1 oz.	1 starch, 2 fat
Vanilla wafers	6 small	1 starch, 1 fat

** If more than one serving is eaten, these foods have 400 mg. or more of sodium.

Free Foods

A free food is any food or drink that contains fewer than 20 calories per serving. You can eat as much as you want of these items that have no serving size specified. You may eat two or three servings per day of those items that have a specific serving size. Be sure to spread them out during the day.

Drinks:

Bouillon
    ** or broth without fat
Bouillon, low-sodium
Carbonated drinks, sugar-free
Carbonated water
Club soda
Cocoa powder, unsweetened (1 tbsp)
Coffee/tea
Drink mixes, sugar-free
Mineral water
Tonic water, sugar-free

Nonstick pan spray

Fruit:

Cranberries, unsweetened (½ cup)
Rhubarb, unsweetened (½ cup)

Vegetables (raw, 1 cup):

Cabbage
Celery
Chinese cabbage *
Cucumber
Green onions
Hot peppers
Mushrooms

Radishes
Zucchini
Salad greens
    Endive
    Escarole
    Lettuce
    Romaine
    Spinach

Sweet Substitutes:

Candy, hard, sugar-free
Gelatin, sugar-free
Gum, sugar-free
Jam/jelly, sugar-free (2 tsp)
Pancake syrup, sugar-free (1/4 cup)
Sugar substitutes (saccharin, aspartame)
Whipped topping (2 tbsp)

Condiments:

Catsup (1 Tbsp)
Horseradish
Mustard
Pickles,** dill unsweetened
Salad dressings, low-calorie (2 Tbsp)
Taco sauce (1 Tbsp)
Vinegar

Seasoning can be very helpful in making food taste better. Be careful of how much sodium you use. Read the label and choose those seasonings which do not contain sodium or salt.*

Basil (fresh)
Celery seeds
Cinnamon

Chili powder
Chives
Curry
Dill
Flavoring extracts (vanilla, lemon, almond, walnut, peppermint, butter, etc.)
Garlic
Garlic powder
Herbs
Hot pepper sauce
Lemon
Lemon juice
Lemon pepper
Lime
Lime juice
Mint
Onion powder
Oregano
Paprika
Pepper
Pimiento
Spices
Soy sauce**
Soy sauce, low sodium ("Lite")
Wine used in cooking (1/4 cup)
Worcestershire sauce

* 3 grams or more of fiber per serving.
** 400 or more milligrams of sodium per serving.

The exchange lists are the basis of a meal planning system designed by a committee of the American Diabetes Association and the American Dietetic Association. While designed primarily for people with diabetes and others who must follow special diets, the exchange lists are based on principles of good nutrition that apply to everyone.
©1986 American Diabetes Association, American Dietetic Association.

Chapter 2
General Information

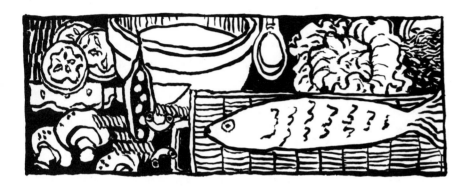

General Information

The majority of recipes in this book have been written to serve 50 portions. Since few kitchens serve exactly 50 portions and many recipes are written for larger portions than needed, it is often necessary to increase or decrease the ingredients in a recipe. When recipes are adjusted it is very important that any changes in the ingredients should be in correct proportion to each other so that the resulting product will be the same as the original.

A WORKING FACTOR is needed to increase or decrease the yield from a recipe. A working factor is established by dividing the number of portions needed by the number of portions in the basic recipe. Most of the recipes in this book yield 50 portions. Therefore, 50 is used as a divisor. If the basic recipe yielded 35 portions, the basic divisor would be 35. If a certain number of servings per pan are specified, the total number of servings would be divided by the number of servings per pan to get the number of pans needed. Then the recipe would be multiplied by the total number of pans needed. It should also be remembered that products such as cakes which should fill the pans 2/3 full of the unbaked batter may need larger or smaller pans than those specified in the original recipe. The size of the pan is very important in the correct preparation of a recipe and the specified pans should always be used, if possible.

TO INCREASE A RECIPE

If 125 portions are needed, the following procedure would be followed:

125 (portions needed) ÷ 50 (portions in basic recipe) = 2.5 (working factor). Since the working factor is 2.5, it will be necessary to increase every ingredient in the recipe 2.5 times. For instance, the recipe for Meat Loaf on page 68 would be increased as follows:

INGREDIENTS	WEIGHTS OR MEASURES X WORKING FACTOR		TOTAL
Eggs	24	× 2.5 = 60	or 5 dz.
Nonfat dry milk	1½ cups	× 2.5 = 3¾ cups	
Very hot water	1 qt.	× 2.5 = 2½ qts.	
Ground lean beef	9 lbs.	× 2.5 = 22	lbs., 8 oz.
Ground lean pork	2 lbs.	× 2.5 = 5	lbs.
Tomato juice	2 cups	× 2.5 = 5	cups or 1¼ qts.
Salt	¼ cup (4 tbsp.)	× 2.5 = 10	tbsp. or ½ cup + 2 tbsp.
Pepper	½ tsp.	× 2.5 = 1¼ tsp.	
Chopped onions	2 cups	× 2.5 = 5	cups or 1¼ qts.
Dry bread crumbs	2 lbs. (2 qts.)	× 2.5 = 5	lbs. or 5 qts. (1¼ gal.)
The yield would also be multiplied	4 loaves	× 2.5 = 10	loaves

TO DECREASE A RECIPE

If 35 portions are needed, the following procedure would be followed:

35 (portions needed) ÷ 50 (portions in basic recipe) = .70.

.70 would be rounded to .75 to get a manageable working factor. (Working factors should generally be divisible by 2, 3 or 4 for ease in converting recipes.) Therefore .75 or ¾ of every ingredient in the recipe would be needed. The meat loaf used to illustrate the preceding recipe increase would be decreased as follows:

INGREDIENTS	WEIGHTS OR MEASURES X WORKING FACTOR		TOTAL
Eggs	24	× .75 = 18	or 1½ dz.
Nonfat dry milk	1½ cups (24 tbsp.)	× .75 = 18	tbsp. or 1 cup + 2 tbsp.
Very hot water	1 qt. (4 cups)	× .75 =	¾ qt. or 3 cups
Lean ground beef	9 lbs.	× .75 = 6¾ lbs.	
Lean ground pork	2 lbs.	× .75 = 1 lbs., 8 oz.	
Tomato juice	2 cups	× .75 = 1½ cups	
Salt	¼ cup (4 tbsp.)	× .75 = 3	tbsp.
Pepper	½ tsp.	× .75 =	¼ tsp. (about)
Chopped onions	2 cups	× .75 = 1½ cups	
Dry bread crumbs	2 lbs. (2 qts.)	× .75 = 1	lb., 8 oz. or (1½ qts.)
The yield would also be multiplied	4 loaves	× .75 = 3	loaves

TO ADAPT A NEW RECIPE

Since many recipes have larger portions than needed, it is often necessary to adapt a new recipe. In order to do this, it is necessary to know how many cups or ounces the recipe yields and how many cups or ounces you need. For instance, if a new recipe yields 50 portions of 6 ounces each and 50 portions of 4 ounces each are needed a working factor would be developed as follows:

50 portions × ½ cup or 4 ounces = 25 cups or 200 ounces needed.

50 portions (new recipe) × ¾ cup or 6 ounces (serving size in new recipe) = 37.5 cups or 300 ounces in new recipe.

200 ounces (amount needed) ÷ 300 ounces (yield of new recipe) = .67 or ⅔ working factor which would be applied to bring the new recipe to the correct size for 50 portions of 4 ounces each.

The working factor would then be applied to decrease the new recipe as illustrated in paragraph above. If the new recipe is smaller than the one needed, it would be increased as illustrated.

EQUIVALENT MEASURES

It is often easier when adapting recipes to use a smaller measure than the one used in the recipe. For instance, the use of cups instead of quarts or teaspoons instead of tablespoons will often make a recipe easier to convert. Measure equivalents to aid in coverting recipes are as follows:

3	tsp.	1 tbsp.
⅛ cup		2 tbsp. or 1 oz.
¼ cup		4 tbsp. or 2 oz.
⅓ cup		5 tbsp. plus 1 tsp.
½ cup		8 tbsp. or 4 oz.
⅔ cup		10 tbsp. plus 2 tsp.
¾ cup		12 tbsp. or 6 oz.
⅞ cup		14 tbsp. or 7 oz.
1	pt.	2 cups
1	lb.	16 oz.
1	qt.	4 cups or 2 pts. or 32 oz.
1	gal.	4 qts. or 16 cups or 128 oz.

It is also often important to know the equivalent measures of certain ingredients when recipes are converted. The following table gives some of the weights and measures used in this book:

ITEM	WEIGHT	APPROX. MEASURES
Meat, Poultry and Fish		
Bacon, chopped cooked	1 pound	5 cups
Bacon, chopped raw	1 pound	3 cups
(1 pound raw bacon yields 4 ounces chopped crisp bacon)		
Chicken or turkey, cubed cooked	1 pound	3 cups
Meat, ground uncooked	1 pound	2 cups
Meat, ground cooked	1 pound	3 cups
Meat, large diced cooked	1 pound	3 cups
Tuna, canned	12½-ounce can	1⅔ cups
Salmon, canned	1 pound can	2 cups
Tuna or salmon, canned	4-pound can	2 quarts
Dairy Foods and Eggs		
Butter	1 pound	2 cups
Cheese, chopped American process	1 pound	4 cups
Cheese, ground American process	1 pound	3 cups
Cheese, shredded or grated Cheddar	1 pound	4 cups
Cheese, cottage	1 pound	2 cups
Cheese, grated Parmesan	4 ounces	1 cup
Cream, sour	1 pound	2 cups
Eggs, medium size, cooked chopped	1 pound	2 cups (6)
Eggs, medium size, raw	1 pound	2 cups (10)
Egg whites, medium size	1 pound	2 cups (16 to 18)
Egg yolks, medium size	1 pound	2 cups (24 to 28)
Egg mix, dehydrated	1 ounce	¼ cup (equal to 2 medium eggs)
Milk, nonfat dry	1 pound	3½ cups
Fruits and Vegetables		
Apples, pared and diced	3½ ounces	1 cup
	1 pound	4¾ cups
Apples, pared and sliced	1 pound	1 quart
Apples, unpared and diced	1 pound	4½ cups
Applesauce, canned	1 pound	1¾ cups
Apricots, dried	1 pound	3 cups
(after cooking)	1 pound 11 ounces	3 cups
Avocados, mashed	1 pound	2 cups

Item	Amount	Equivalent
Bananas, fresh	1 pound	3 medium
Bananas, mashed	1 pound	2 cups (6 medium)
Bananas, sliced	1 pound	3⅓ cups
Bean sprouts, drained canned	1 pound	4½ cups
Beans, dry kidney	1 pound	2½ cups
Beans, dry lima	1 pound	2⅓ cups
Beans, dry pinto	1 pound	2½ cups
Beans, dry white	1 pound	2⅓ cups
Blueberries, frozen	1 pound	3 cups
Boysenberries, frozen	1 pound	3¾ cups
Cabbage, chopped or shredded raw (loose)	1 pound	1¾ quarts
Cabbage, chopped very fine raw	1 pound	5 cups
Carrots, diced raw	1 pound	3½ cups
Carrots, ground or shredded raw	1 pound	1 quart
Carrots, sliced ¼-inch raw	1 pound	3 cups
Cauliflower, flowerettes raw	1 pound	5 cups
Celery, chopped or diced fresh	1 pound	3 cups
Celery, ¾-inch diagonal slice raw	1 pound	4½ cups
Celery, ½-inch pieces raw	1 pound	1 quart
Cranberries, fresh	1 pound	1 quart
Cranberry sauce, all textures	1 pound	1¾ cups
Cucumbers, pared and diced, fresh	1 pound	1 quart
Cucumbers, pared and finely diced, fresh	1 pound	2½ cups
Cucumbers, pared sliced ⅛-inch, fresh	1 pound	3 cups
Currants, dried	1 pound	3 cups
Dates, pitted	1 pound	3 cups
Dates, pitted, chopped	1 pound	3½ cups
Endive, torn, fresh	1 pound	3¼ quarts
Escarole, torn, fresh	1 pound	1 gallon
Fruit mix, candied	1 pound	2 cups
Garlic, minced	1 clove	1 teaspoon
(1 clove dry garlic equals ¼ teaspoon dehydrated garlic)		
Grapes, seeded and cut, fresh	1 pound	2¾ cups
Honeydew melon balls, fresh	3 pounds A.P.	1 quart balls / 24 ounces E.P.
Lemons for juice, fresh	1 lemon (4 ounces)	2 tbsp. juice
Lemon rind, grated	1 ounce	⅓ cup (8 lemons)
Lettuce, shredded, packed	1 pound	1 quart
Lettuce, torn fresh, not packed	1 pound	2½ quarts
Onions, chopped dry	1 pound	3 cups
Onions, minced dry	1 pound	2⅔ cups
Onions, thinly sliced dry	1 pound	3 cups
Onions, green, chopped with tops	1 pound	5⅓ cups
Orange sections, fresh	1 pound	2 cups
Oranges for juice	1 pound	½ cup juice (2)
Orange rind	1 ounce	3 tbsp. 1 large orange
Parsley, chopped or minced fresh	2 ounces	1 cup
Parsley, dehydrated	1½ ounce	1 cup
Peas, split, green, dry	1 pound	2 cups
Peppers, dehydrated green	1 ounce	¾ cup
Peppers, sweet chopped green	1 pound	3 cups
Peppers, sweet minced green	1 pound	2⅔ cups
Pimientos, chopped drained	1 pound	2 cups
Potatoes, cooked or raw, ½-inch diced	1 pound	3 cups
Potatoes, cooked, mashed	1 pound	2 cups
Prunes, dried, 40 to 50 size	1 pound	2½ cups
Prunes, dried, 30 to 40 size	1 pound	3½ cups
Radishes, sliced thin	1 pound	3 cups
Radishes, cleaned and trimmed	1 pound	1 quart
Raisins, seedless	1 pound	3 cups
Rhubarb, 1-inch pieces raw	1 pound	1 quart (2½ cups cooked)
Romaine, cut up fresh	1 pound	2½ quarts
Sauerkraut, canned	1 pound	2 cups
Spinach, raw	1 pound	1 gallon
Strawberries, frozen	1 pound	2 cups
Tomatoes, diced fresh	1 pound	2¾ cups
Tomato wedges, fresh	1 pound	3¼ cups
Turnips, diced raw	1 pound	3½ cups

Bakery and Cereal Products

Barley, pearl	1 pound	2 cups
Bread crumbs, finely ground dry	1 pound	1 quart
Bread crumbs, soft fresh	1 pound	1¼ quarts
Bread, sliced	1 pound	16 slices
Cake crumbs	1 pound	1 quart
Cornflake crumbs	1 pound	1 quart
Cereal, rolled oats	1 pound	1½ quarts (9 cups cooked)
Cornmeal	1 pound	2¾ cups
Crackers, graham	1 pound	64-66 crackers
Cracker crumbs, graham	1 pound	1 quart
Cracker crumbs, soda	1 pound	6½ cups
Flour, wheat, all-purpose sifted	1 pound	1 quart
Flour, wheat, all-purpose unsifted	18 ounces	1 quart
Hominy grits, dry	1 pound	2⅔ cups
Macaroni, elbow, dry	1 pound	4 cups
1 pound after it is cooked	3 lbs	
	2½ ounces	9 cups
Macaroni, medium dry shells	1 pound	5½ cups
Noodles, dry	1 pound	1½ quart
1 pound after it is cooked	3⅔ pounds	2¼ quart
Pancake mix	1 pound	3⅓ cups
Rice, instant dry	1 pound	4¾ cups
Rice, long grain	1 pound	2¼ cups
Rice, milled, dry	1 pound	2⅓ cups
1 pound after it is cooked	3½ pounds	2 quarts
Spaghetti, 2-inch pieces, dry	1 pound	2 quarts
Starch, cornstarch	1 pound	3¼ cups
	1 ounce	3 tbsp.
Tapioca, minute	1 pound	2⅔ cups

Sugar, Confectionary and Nuts

Almond paste	1 pound	1¾ cups
Chocolate, semisweet cooking	6 ounces	1 cup
Chocolate chips	6 ounces	1 cup
Coconut, chopped	8 ounces	2¾ cups
Coconut, flaked	3 ounces	1 cup
Honey	12 ounces	1 cup
Marshmallows, miniature	1 pound	9 cups
Molasses	12 ounces	1 cup
Nuts, chopped	1 pound	1 quart
Sugar, packed brown	7½ ounces	1 cup
	1 pound	2¾ cups
Sugar, sifted powdered	1 pound	1 quart
Sugar, unsifted powdered	1 pound	3½ cups
Sugar, granulated	1 pound	2¼ cups
Syrup, blended corn and refiners	11½ ounces	1 cup
	1 pound	1⅓ cups

Jams, Jellies and Preserves

Jams, fruit	2 pounds	2¾ cups
Peanut butter	9 ounces	1 cup
	1 pound	1¾ cups
Jelly	10 ounces	1 cup
	1 pound	1½ cups

Soup and gravy base, beef, chicken or ham flavor

	1 ounce	3 tbsp.
	1 pound	3 cups

Edible Oils and Fats

Margarine	1 pound	2 cups
Salad oil	15 ounces	2 cups
Shortening	1 pound	2¼ cups
	7¼ ounces	1 cup

Condiments and Related Products

Allspice, ground	1 ounce	4 tbsp.
Baking powder	1 ounce	2¼ tbsp.
Baking soda	1 ounce	2½ tbsp.
Basil, sweet ground	1 ounce	6 tbsp.
Caraway seed	1 ounce	3 tbsp.
Catsup	10 ounces	1 cup
	1 pound	1⅔ cups
Celery seed	1 ounce	4 tbsp.
Chili powder	1 ounce	4 tbsp.
Chili sauce	1 pound	1½ cups
Cinnamon, ground	1 ounce	4 tbsp.
Cloves, ground	1 ounce	4 tbsp.
Cloves, whole	1 ounce	5 tbsp.
Cocoa	1 pound	1 quart
	4 ounces	1 cup

Cream of tartar	1 ounce	3 tbsp.
Gelatin, fruit-flavored	1 pound	2⅓ cups
Gelatin, fruit-flavored	7 ounces	1 cup
Ginger, ground	1 ounce	4 tbsp.
Horseradish, prepared	1 pound	1½ cups
Lemon extract	1 ounce	2⅓ tbsp.
Mace, ground	1 ounce	4½ tbsp.
Mustard, ground	1 ounce	5 tbsp.
Mustard, salad	1 ounce	2 tbsp.
	1 pound	2 cups
Nutmeg, ground	1 ounce	4 tbsp.
Olives, pitted, sliced	4 ounces	1 cup
Oregano, ground	1 ounce	5 tbsp.
Paprika, ground	1 ounce	4 tbsp.
Pepper, black or cayenne, ground	1 ounce	4 tbsp.
Pickles, chopped	1 pound	2½ cups
Poppyseed	1 ounce	3 tbsp.
Poultry seasoning, ground	1 ounce	4 tbsp.
Relish, sweet pickle	1 pound	2 cups
Sage, ground	1 ounce	½ cup
Salad dressing	1 pound	2 cups
Salt	1 pound	1½ cups
	1 ounce	1½ tbsp.
Sesame seed	1 ounce	3 tbsp.
Thyme, ground	1 ounce	6 tbsp.
Vanilla	1 ounce	2 tbsp.
Vinegar	1 pound	2 cups
Yeast, active dry	1 ounce	3 tbsp.
Cocoa beverage powder	1 pound	2⅔ cups
Coffee, instant	2 ounces	1 cup
Coffee, roasted ground	1 pound	5 cups
Ice, crushed or cubed	4 pounds	1 gallon
Tea, loose black	2 ounces	¾ cup

* Data in this table is based upon information furnished by The Ration Design and Evaluation Branch, U.S. Army, Natick, Research and Development Center, Natick, Mass. 01760.

NONFAT DRY MILK

Many of the recipes in this book specify nonfat dry milk because it is easy to use, easy to store and economical. Nonfat dry milk can be kept in its original container or in a covered canister in a cool dry place along with other staples. It does not need to be refrigerated until after it has been reconstituted by the addition of water. For general cooking purposes, nonfat dry milk should be reconstituted by stirring it into warm water. It should be refrigerated after it is reconstituted unless it is to be used immediately. Whenever possible, the nonfat dry milk should be combined with the other ingredients and water added as a liquid.

Children and older people particularly benefit from the use of nonfat dry milk because it can be used to enrich their food with additional protein, minerals and vitamins in foods which do not ordinarily contain as much milk.

The following table of milk equivalents may be used for the substitution of nonfat dry milk in recipes which use liquid skim milk.

Reconstitution of Nonfat Dry Milk

NONFAT DRY MILK +	WATER =	FLUID SKIM MILK
6 tablespoons	1⅞ cups	2 cups
¾ cup	3¾ cups	1 quart
1½ cups	1 quart, 3½ cups	2 quarts
2¼ cups	2¾ quarts	3 quarts
3 cups	3¾ quarts	1 gallon
1½ quarts	1 gallon, 3½ quarts	2 gallons
2¼ quarts	2 gallons, 3¼ quarts	3 gallons
3 quarts	3¾ gallons	4 gallons
3¾ quarts	4¾ gallons	5 gallons

NONFAT DRY MILK +	WATER + Added fat =	FLUID WHOLE MILK
1½ tablespoons	½ cup	½ cup
3 tablespoons	⅞ cup	1 cup
6 tablespoons (1¾ ounces)	1⅞ cups	2 cups
¾ cup (3¼ ounces)	3¾ cups, 2 tablespoons	1 quart
1½ cups (6½ ounces)	7½ cups, 5 tablespoons	2 quarts
3 cups (13 ounces)	3¾ quarts, ⅔ cup	1 gallon
4 pounds, 1 ounce		
3½ quarts	4⅔ gallons, 3 cups	5 gallons

INSTANT NONFAT DRY MILK does not have the same volume as regular nonfat dry milk and cannot be substituted for regular nonfat dry milk on a measure-for-measure basis. If it is necessary to use instant nonfat dry milk instead of the regular nonfat dry milk, it should be done on a pound-for-pound basis, figuring that 1 ounce of regular nonfat dry milk measures 3½ tablespoons and 4½ ounces of regular nonfat dry milk measures 1 cup.

PURCHASING

Efficient purchasing of food is very important in good kitchen management. It helps prevent leftover food and helps keep the cost per portion at a reasonable level. Recipes in this book can be used as a purchasing guide for meat and many other items. However, such items as carrots, onions, etc., which are commonly kept on hand do not have weights specified in the recipes. The following table has been included as a help for purchasing those items. The table shows how much peeled or prepared food you can expect from the purchase of 1 pound of raw weight of a specified item.

INGREDIENT	EDIBLE PORTION IN 1 LB. AS PURCHASED
Apples, whole	3 to 4 medium
Apples, diced for salad	2¾ cups
Bananas, whole	3 medium
Bananas, sliced	2¼ cups
Cabbage, shredded	1½ qts.
Carrots, chopped or sliced	3 to 3¼ cups
Celery, sliced	2½ to 3 cups
Cucumbers, sliced	2½ to 3 cups
Lettuce, whole	12 oz.
Lettuce, shredded	3 cups
Onions, chopped	2½ to 3 cups
Onions, sliced	3½ to 4 cups
Fresh green peppers, chopped	2½ to 3 cups
Potatoes, white, peeled	13 oz.
Radishes, trimmed	1 qt.
Radishes, sliced	3 cups
Tomatoes, fresh, whole	3 to 4 medium
Tomatoes, trimmed	14 to 14½ oz.
Tomatoes, sliced	2½ cups
Turnips, peeled, diced	2¼ cups
Endive	1 gal.
Escarole	1 gal.
Romaine	2½ qts.

Frozen and canned fruit juices are a very important part of the daily diet. Frozen juices should be kept in the freezer at 0°F. or lower and canned fruit juices should be kept in a cool, airy storeroom. Yields from juices may be figured as follows:

Canned and Frozen Fruit Juices

TYPE OF JUICE	SIZE OF CONTAINER	YIELD
Frozen Orange Juice (3 plus 1)	32-oz. can	32 4-oz. juice glasses
	12-oz. can	12 4-oz. juice glasses
Canned Juices (single strength)	No. 10 can	24 4-oz. juice glasses
	No. 3 cyl. can	11 4-oz. juice glasses

It is also important when purchasing foods to recognize the common can sizes, their capacity and how many are packed in a case.

Common Case Sizes

CAN SIZE	AVERAGE WEIGHT AND MEASURE	CANS PER CASE
No. 10	6 lbs. 8 oz., 12 to 13 cups	6
No. 3 cycl.	3 lbs. 3 oz., 5¾ cups	12
No. 2½	1 lb. 11 oz., 3½ cups	24
No. 2	1 lb. 4 oz., 2½ cups	24
No. 303	16 or 17 oz., 2 cups	24 or 36
No. 300	14 to 16 oz., 1¾ cups	24
No. 1 (picnic)	10½ to 12 oz., 1¼ cups	48
8 oz.	8 oz., 1 cup	48 or 72

If it is necessary to substitute one can size for another, the following table can be used as a guide:

Can Substitutions

CAN SIZE	NUMBER OF CANS TO USE IN PLACE OF A No. 10 CAN	CONTENTS OF EACH CAN
No. 3 Cyl.	2	5¾ cups
No. 2½	4	3½ cups
No. 2	5	2½ cups
No. 303	7	2 cups

DIPPERS AND LADLES

Dipper numbers are based on the number of level dippers in 1 quart. For instance, a No. 16 dipper is 1/16 of a quart of 1/4 of a cup. Ladle numbers refer to the number of ounces a ladle will hold. For instance, an 8 ounce ladle holds 8 ounces or 1 cup. All measures are level. Some of the more commonly used dippers and ladles are as follows:

Dipper Sizes

NUMBER	MEASURES (APPROXIMATE)	WEIGHT (APPROXIMATE)
60	1 tbsp.	1/2 oz.
40	1½ tbsp.	3/4 oz.
24	2¾ tbsp.	1½ oz. to 1¾ oz.
20	3 tbsp.	1¾ oz. to 2 oz.
16	4 tbsp., 1/4 cup	2 oz.
12	5 tbsp., 1/3 cup	2½ oz. to 3 oz.
10	6 tbsp.	3 oz. to 4 oz.
8	8 tbsp., 1/2 cup	4 oz.
6	10 tbsp.	5 oz.

Ladle Sizes

NUMBER	CAPACITY
1 oz.	2 tbsp., 1/8 cup
2 oz.	4 tbsp., 1/4 cup
4 oz.	8 tbsp., 1/2 cup
6 oz.	12 tbsp., 3/4 cup
8 oz.	16 tbsp., 1 cup

MEASURES

All measures in this book are level, and it is emphasized that the correct number of portions cannot be served from a recipe unless all measures and portions are level. Weight and/or measures have been used for various foods according to the most commonly used measurements of that food.

Flour should not be sifted unless the directions specify sifting since there is a difference in the measurements for sifted and unsifted flour. Flour should be scooped lightly into a measure and leveled with a straight-edged knife or spatula. It should never be shaken to level it because this will result in an increased amount of flour in the measure.

EQUIPMENT

The simplest equipment has been used in directions for these recipes. However, it is presumed that all kitchens have institutional-size mixers and standard cooking and baking equipment. If possible, it is recommended that all kitchens have a convection oven, institutional-type food processor and steamer as well as adequate refrigeration and freezing units.

Convection ovens are recommended because they save time and energy since they bake at a lower temperature and in a shorter time than the conventional ovens.

Food processors are recommended because they save so much time in food preparation. If possible, they should have a continuous feed attachment for even greater time savings.

Steamers save time, yield a better produce and help preserve nutrients in fruits and vegetables cooked in the steamer.

Adequate refrigeration is necessary for the preservation of food and adequate freezer space makes it possible to purchase food in larger quantities and to serve a greater variety of food.

When new equipment is purchased, instructions which come with the equipment should be studied thoroughly and then filed for future use if the item needs to be repaired. Most manufacturers will send a representative to explain use of new large equipment and it is always wise to take advantage of this service in order to use the equipment more efficiently.

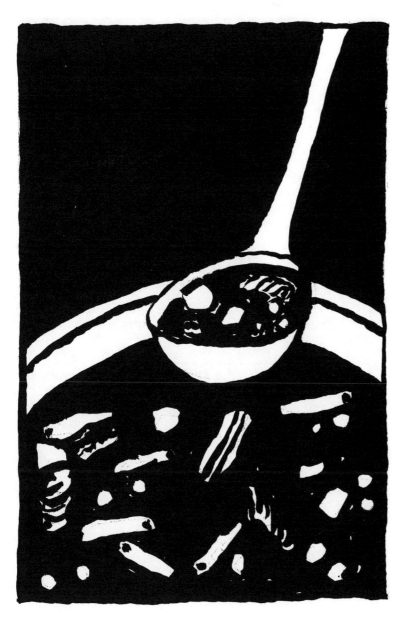

Chapter 3
Soups

YIELD
50 portions (about 2½ gallons)

PAN SIZE
Heavy 5-gallon pot

PORTION SIZE
¾ cup (6-ounce ladle)

DIETARY INFORMATION
May be used as written for general, no added salt and mechanical soft diets. Diabetic diets — each serving provides 1 bread and 1 lean meat exchanges. Bland diets — omit pepper. Each serving provides 1 ounce meat equivalent.

Bean Soup

Refer to footnotes for special dietary information

INGREDIENTS	WEIGHTS/MEASURES	YIELD ADJUST.	METHOD
Dry white beans . . . . .2 pounds, 8 ounces (1½ quarts) Cold water. . . . . .3 quarts			1. Pick over beans and remove any foreign matter; wash beans thoroughly in cold water. 2. Cover beans with 3 quarts cold water; bring to a boil; cook 2 minutes. Turn off heat; let beans stand 1 to 2 hours.
Ham stock. . . . . .2½ gallons			3. Add stock which has been chilled, the fat removed and strained, to the beans. (Prepare ham stock with ham soup base according to directions on the container, if ham bones are not available.) Bring to a boil, cover and simmer 1½ hours or until beans are tender.
Shredded carrots . . . . .1½ cups Finely chopped onions. . . . . . .1½ cups Pepper. . . . . .1 teaspoon Diced cooked ham . . . . .1 pound			4. Add carrots, onions and pepper to beans; simmer 30 minutes; add ham.
All-purpose flour. . . . . .1 cup Cold water. . . . . .1½ cups			5. Mix flour and water together until smooth; stir mixture into soup; cook another 10 minutes, stirring occasionally. Serve hot.

Cheese Soup

Refer to footnotes for special dietary information

INGREDIENTS WEIGHTS/MEASURES	YIELD ADJUST.	METHOD
Finely chopped carrots......1¼ cups Finely chopped celery ....1¼ cups Finely chopped onions......1¼ cups Margarine or chicken fat......1 cup		1. Fry vegetables in the pot for 5 minutes in margarine or chicken fat, stirring occasionally. 2. Take vegetables out of the fat with a slotted spoon; put vegetables aside for use in step 4.
Cornstarch ....⅓ cup All-purpose flour............1 cup Paprika ....1 teaspoon White pepper..............1 teaspoon Salt ....1 tablespoon		3. Mix cornstarch, flour, paprika, pepper and salt together. Stir flour mixture into fat; cook and stir over moderate heat 3 to 4 minutes or until smooth.
Cold chicken stock.........1½ gallons		4. Add chicken stock to flour mixture; cook and stir until smooth; simmer 10 minutes, stirring occasionally; add cooked vegetables.
Nonfat dry milk.............1¼ quarts Warm water...............3 quarts Shredded or chopped cheddar or American process cheese 12 ounces Chopped parsley (optional)		5. Stir dry milk into warm water; add with cheese to the soup just before serving. Heat soup slowly to serving temperature but do not let it boil. (Cheese should be dissolved in the soup.) 6. Garnish soup with chopped parsley. Serve hot.

YIELD
50 portions (about 2½ gallons)

PORTION SIZE
¾ cup (6-ounce ladle)

PAN SIZE
Heavy 5-gallon pot

DIETARY INFORMATION
May be used as written for general, no added salt and mechanical soft diets. Diabetic diets — each serving provides ½ bread and 1 fat exchanges. Bland diets — omit pepper.

YIELD
50 portions (about 2½ gallons)

PORTION SIZE
¾ cup (6-ounce ladle)

PAN SIZE
Heavy 5-gallon pot

DIETARY INFORMATION
May be used as written for general, no added salt and mechanical soft diets. Diabetic diets — each serving provides 1 bread, 1 fat and ½ vegetable exchanges. Bland diet — omit pepper and fresh green peppers. Low cholesterol diets — omit bacon. Use ¼ cup vegetable oil in step 1.

Corn Chowder

Refer to footnotes for special dietary information

INGREDIENTS	WEIGHTS/MEASURES	YIELD ADJUST.	METHOD
Chopped bacon ....8 ounces Chopped celery.............½ cup Chopped onions ....1½ cups Chopped fresh green peppers .¾ cup			1. Fry bacon in pot until it is crisp; add celery, onions and green peppers and cook 7 minutes, stirring occasionally.
Chicken stock.............3 quarts Diced fresh white potatoes....1 quart Salt ....2½ tablespoons White pepper..............½ teaspoon			2. Add chicken stock, potatoes, salt and pepper to bacon mixture; simmer 15 minutes or until potatoes are tender.
Cream-style corn...........3 quarts (1 No. 10 can)			3. Add corn to soup; bring to a boil and cook 5 minutes, stirring occasionally.
Nonfat dry milk............1¼ quarts Warm water...............3 quarts Margarine ....¾ cup (1½ sticks)			4. Stir dry milk into warm water; add warm milk and margarine to soup; heat slowly to serving temperature but do not boil; serve hot.

Fish Chowder

Refer to footnotes for special dietary information

INGREDIENTS	WEIGHTS/MEASURES	YIELD ADJUST.	METHOD
Skinless fish fillets, cut in 1/2-inch pieces . . . . .4 pounds Diced fresh white potatoes. . . .1 quart Boiling water. . . . . .1 gallon			1. Add fish and potatoes to water; simmer 20 minutes or until potatoes are tender.
Diced bacon . . . . .8 ounces			2. Fry bacon until crisp; remove bacon from fat with a slotted spoon; add bacon to fish mixture.
Finely chopped onions . . . . . . .2 1/2 cups			3. Fry onions in bacon fat until golden.
Margarine . . . . .1 cup (8 ounces) All-purpose flour . . . . .2 cups			4. Add margarine and flour to onions and bacon fat; cook and stir until smooth; set aside for use in step 6.
Nonfat dry milk . . . . .1 quart Warm water. . . . . .1 gallon			5. Stir milk into warm water; add milk to fish and potatoes; heat to just below boiling point but do not boil.
Salt . . . . .2 1/2 tablespoons White pepper. . . . . .1 teaspoon			6. Add flour mixture to soup; stir to mix well; simmer 1/2 hour to thicken soup and improve flavor; add salt and pepper; serve hot.

YIELD
50 portions (about 2 1/2 gallons)

PORTION SIZE
3/4 cup (6-ounce ladle)

PAN SIZE
Heavy 5-gallon pot

DIETARY INFORMATION
May be used as written for general, no added salt and mechanical soft diets. Diabetic diets — each serving provides 1/2 bread, 1 lean meat and 1 fat exchanges. Bland diets — omit pepper. Each serving provides 1 ounce fish.

YIELD
50 portions (about 2¼ gallons)

PORTION SIZE
¾ cup (6-ounce ladle)

PAN SIZE
Heavy 3-gallon pot

DIETARY INFORMATION
May be used as written for general, bland, and no added salt diets. For low cholesterol, omit sour cream. Diabetic diets — omit sugar. Use water in step 1. Use unsweetened canned pineapple in step 3. Sweeten to taste with sugar substitute at the end of step 3. Served without whipped topping, each serving provides ½ bread and 1 fruit exchanges.

Fruit Soup

Refer to footnotes for special dietary information

INGREDIENTS	WEIGHTS/MEASURES	YIELD ADJUST.	METHOD
Chopped pitted prunes.......2 pounds Golden raisins..............2 cups Sugar.....................3 cups Cold water.................2 gallons Stick cinnamon............4 sticks			1. Place prunes, raisins, sugar, water and stick cinnamon in pot. Cover and simmer 30 minutes over low heat. Remove cinnamon sticks from the soup. (Fruit juice may be used instead of water. If fruit juice is used, the amount of sugar should be adjusted according to the sweetness of the juice.)
Cornstarch ....½ cup Cold water.................1 cup Lemon juice ....½ cup Frozen orange juice concentrate.............2 cups			2. Dissolve cornstarch in water and stir until smooth. Add, along with lemon and orange juices, to the soup. Cook and stir over moderate heat until slightly thickened and the starchy taste is gone.
Drained canned pineapple tidbits ....1 quart Sour cream (optional) ....3 cups Whipped topping (optional) ...3 cups			3. Add pineapple to soup. Mix lightly. Reheat, if necessary. Serve hot as a first course garnished with 1 tablespoon sour cream or cold as a dessert garnished with 1 tablespoon whipped topping, or use as a topping over ice cream.

Goulash Soup

Refer to footnotes for special dietary information

INGREDIENTS	WEIGHTS/MEASURES	YIELD ADJUST.	METHOD

Chopped onions . . . . .2 quarts
Vegetable oil . . . . .½ cup
Beef round, trimmed of
   all fat and cut into
   ½-inch cubes . . . . .4 pounds
			1. Cook and stir onions in ¼ cup oil in pot over moderate heat until onions are limp. Remove onions with a slotted spoon and set aside for use in step 2.
			2. Add remaining oil to pot and brown beef in hot oil over medium heat, stirring frequently. Return onions to pot.

Fat-free beef broth . . . . .2½ gallons Garlic powder . . . . .1 tablespoon Paprika . . . . .3 tablespoons Drained canned crushed tomatoes. . . . . .1 quart Salt . . . . .as necessary			3. Add broth, garlic, paprika and tomatoes to meat. Cover and simmer about 1 hour or until meat is tender. Taste for seasoning and add more salt, if necessary. (The amount of salt necessary will depend upon the saltiness of the broth.)
Cubed fresh white potatoes . . .2 quarts			4. Add potatoes to soup. Cover and simmer 15 to 20 minutes or until potatoes are tender. Serve hot.

SOUPS 6

YIELD
50 portions (about 3 gallons)

PORTION SIZE
1 cup (8-ounce ladle)

PAN SIZE
Heavy 5-gallon pot

DIETARY INFORMATION
May be used as written for general, bland and no added salt diets. Diabetic diets — each serving provides 1 lean meat and 1 vegetable exchanges. Low cholesterol diets — trim all visible fat from beef. Each serving provides 1 ounce beef.

YIELD
50 portions (about 2¼ gallons)

PORTION SIZE
¾ cup (6-ounce ladle)

PAN SIZE
Heavy 3-gallon pot

DIETARY INFORMATION
May be used as written for general, no added salt and mechanical soft diets. Diabetic diets — each serving provides 1 lean meat and 1 bread exchanges. Bland diets — omit pepper. Low cholesterol diets — use baked ham from which all visible fat has been removed. Each serving provides 1 ounce meat.

Ham and Yam Chowder

Refer to footnotes for special dietary information

INGREDIENTS	WEIGHTS/MEASURES	YIELD ADJUST.	METHOD
Smoked boneless pork shoulder cut in ½-inch cubes or Trimmings from baked ham, cut in bite-size pieces . . . . . . 4 pounds, 4 ounces (about 3 quarts) Hot water . . . . 1½ gallons			1. Fry ham in pot over moderate heat, stirring occasionally, for about 5 minutes or until lightly browned; add hot water; cover and simmer 30 minutes for smoked, boneless, pork shoulder or 15 minutes for ham trimmings.
Fresh yams . . . . 5 pounds Drained cooked whole kernel corn . . . . 2 quarts Salt . . . . as necessary Pepper . . . . ½ teaspoon			2. Peel yams; cut into about ½-inch cubes; add yams and corn to ham; cover and simmer about 20 minutes or until yams are tender; add salt to taste and pepper. (The amount of salt needed will depend upon the saltiness of the ham.)
All-purpose flour . . . . 1 cup Nonfat dry milk . . . . 1 cup Cold water . . . . 1 quart			3. Add flour and dry milk to cold water; stir until smooth; add slowly to soup; cook and stir over moderate heat until smooth; continue to cook, stirring occasionally, over low heat about 5 minutes or until the starchy taste is gone. Serve hot.

Hamburger Soup

Refer to footnotes for special dietary information

INGREDIENTS	WEIGHTS/MEASURES	YIELD ADJUST.	METHOD
Lean ground beef . . . . .4 pounds, 8 ounces			1. Place beef in preheated frying pan. Cook and stir in its own fat, over moderate heat, until meat is separated and browned. 2. Place meat in colander and drain well. Discard fat and liquid. Place meat in pot.
Fat-free beef broth . . . . .2 ¼ gallons Chopped onions . . . . .2 quarts			3. Add broth and onions to meat. Cover and simmer 20 minutes. Skim off any fat which has risen to the top of the soup.
Frozen peas and carrots . . . . . .3 quarts (6 pounds) Quick-cooking barley . . . . .1 cup Thyme . . . . .1 teaspoon White pepper (optional) . . . . . .1 teaspoon Salt .3 to 4 tablespoons			4. Add peas and carrots, barley, thyme, pepper and salt to the soup. (The amount of salt necessary will depend upon the saltiness of the broth.) Cover and simmer 20 minutes.
Instant potatoes or potato buds . . . . .2 cups			5. Stir potatoes into the soup. Cover and continue to simmer for another 5 minutes.
Sour cream . . . . .1 quart Chopped parsley . . . . .as necessary			6. Stir 1 quart of the hot soup into the sour cream. Remove the soup from the heat and stir the sour cream mixture back into the soup. Reheat the soup, if necessary, but do not let it come to a boil after the sour cream is added. 7. Serve the soup hot with a garnish of parsley.

YIELD
50 portions (about 3 gallons)

PORTION SIZE
1 cup (8-ounce ladle)

PAN SIZE
Heavy frying pan
Heavy 5-gallon pot

DIETARY INFORMATION
May be used as written for general, no added salt and mechanical soft diets. Diabetic diets — each serving as written provides 2 lean meat, 1 bread and 1 fat exchanges. Each serving without the sour cream provides 2 lean meat and 1 bread exchanges. Bland diets — omit pepper. Low cholesterol diets — omit sour cream. Use 2 15½-ounce cans of evaporated skim milk or serve plain without cream or milk. Each serving provides 1 ounce of meat.

YIELD
50 portions (about 3 gallons)

PORTION SIZE
1 cut (8-ounce ladle)

PAN SIZE
Heavy 5-gallon pot

DIETARY INFORMATION
May be used as written for general and no added salt diets. Diabetic diets — each serving provides 2½ bread and 1 lean meat exchanges. Bland diets — omit fresh green peppers and pepper. Low cholesterol diets — remove all visible fat from ham. Each serving provides 2 ounces meat and equivalents.

Lentil Soup

Refer to footnotes for special dietary information

INGREDIENTS	WEIGHTS/MEASURES	YIELD ADJUST.	METHOD
Chopped onions . . . . .1 quart Chopped celery. . . . . .1 quart Chopped fresh green peppers .2 cups Vegetable oil . . . . .¼ cup			1. Cook and stir onions, celery and peppers in oil in pot until onions are limp.
Hot fat-free ham stock . . . . . . .3 gallons Ham scraps. . . . . .1½ quarts 　　　　　　　　　　　(2 pounds) Dried lentils. . . . . .6 pounds 　　　　　　　　　　(about 3½ quarts) Catsup . . . . .2 cups Molasses . . . . .½ cup Vinegar . . . . .½ cup Dry mustard . . . . .1 tablespoon Salt . . . . .as necessary			2. Add stock, ham, lentils, catsup, molasses, vinegar and mustard to vegetables in pot. Cover and simmer for 2 hours or until lentils are tender and beginning to fall apart. 3. Taste for seasoning and add more salt, if necessary. (The amount of salt necessary will depend upon the saltiness of the stock.) Serve hot.

Minestrone

Refer to footnotes for special dietary information

INGREDIENTS	WEIGHTS/MEASURES	YIELD ADJUST.	METHOD
Dry beans . . . . .2 pounds (4²/₃ cups) Beef broth . . . . .2³/₄ gallons			1. Pick over the beans; remove any dirt or discolored beans; wash beans thoroughly in cold water; drain. 2. Put beans in pot; add beef broth; boil 2 minutes; remove from heat; cover and let stand 1 to 2 hours. 3. Bring beans and broth to a boil; reduce heat and simmer 1 hour.
Diced bacon . . . . .8 ounces Finely chopped onions . . . . . .2 cups Finely chopped celery . . . . . . .1 cup			4. Fry bacon until crisp; add onions and celery and continue to cook until onions are golden; add to beans.
Dried parsley. . . . . .¹/₄ cup Chopped frozen green beans . .1 pound (1 quart) Diced fresh white potatoes. . . .2 cups Canned pear tomatoes. . . . . . .3¹/₂ cups (1 No. 2¹/₂ can) Finely diced carrots . . . . .¹/₂ cup Finely diced cabbage . . . . .2 cups Minced garlic cloves. . . . . .6 Pepper. . . . . .¹/₂ teaspoon Italian seasoning . . . . .2 tablespoons Leaf oregano. . . . . .1 tablespoon Basil .1 teaspoon			5. Add parsley, green beans, potatoes, tomatoes, carrots, cabbage, garlic, pepper, Italian seasoning, oregano and basil to beans; continue to simmer another 2 hours or until beans are mushy; break up some of the beans against the side of the pot with the back of a large spoon.
Diced cooked beef . . . . .2 pounds, 10 ounces Water. . . . . .as necessary Macaroni or spaghetti . . . . . . .12 ounces Salt . . . . .to taste Grated Parmesan cheese . . . . .1 pound			6. Add diced beef to soup; add more water to the soup, if necessary, to bring the volume back to 2¹/₂ gallons. Bring the soup back to a boil; add macaroni or spaghetti. (Break the spaghetti into bite-size pieces, if spaghetti is used.) Cook 12 to 15 minutes or until macaroni or spaghetti is tender. Add salt to taste; serve hot; garnish with grated cheese using about 1 tablespoon per serving.

YIELD
50 portions (about 2¹/₂ gallons)

PORTION SIZE
³/₄ cup (6-ounce ladle)

PAN SIZE
Heavy 5-gallon pot

DIETARY INFORMATION
May be used as written for general, no added salt and mechanical soft diets. Diabetic diets — each serving as written provides 1 vegetable, 1 bread and 2 lean meat exchanges. Each serving without the spaghetti and cheese provides 1 bread and 1 lean meat exchanges. Bland diets — omit peppers. Low cholesterol diets — omit bacon. Use ¹/₄ cup vegetable oil in step 4. Remove all visible fat from beef in step 6. Each serving provides 2 ounces of meat and equivalent.

YIELD
50 portions (about 3 gallons)

PORTION SIZE
1 cup (8 ounce ladle)

PAN SIZE
Heavy 5-gallon pot

DIETARY INFORMATION
May be used as written for general, no salt and low cholesterol diets. Diabetic diets — the recipe as written provides per serving 1 lean meat and 1/2 bread exchanges. The recipe without rice provides per serving 1 lean meat, 1 vegetable and 1 fat exchanges. Bland diets — omit curry powder, cloves and pepper. Each serving provides 1 ounce chicken or turkey.

Mulligatawny Soup

Refer to footnotes for special dietary information

INGREDIENTS	WEIGHTS/MEASURES	YIELD ADJUST.	METHOD
Chopped onions . . . . .2 cups Diced carrots . . . . .2 cups Diced celery . . . . .2 cups Margarine . . . . .1/4 cup			1. Place onions, carrots, celery and margarine in pot. Cook and stir over medium heat until onions are limp.

Hot fat-free chicken broth. . . . .2 1/4 gallons
Chopped drained canned
   tomatoes. . . . . .1 1/2 quarts
Diced or sliced cored tart
   apples . . . . .3 cups
Curry powder . . . . .2 teaspoons
Ground cloves. . . . . .1/2 teaspoon
Salt . . . . .2 teaspoons
White pepper (optional). . . . . .1/2 teaspoon
			2. Add broth, tomatoes, apples and seasonings to vegetables. Cover and simmer 45 minutes. Test for seasoning and add more salt, if necessary. (The amount of salt needed will depend upon the saltiness of the broth.)

All-purpose flour . . . . .2 cups Cool fat-free chicken broth . . . .1 quart			3. Make a smooth paste with the flour and broth. Stir into the simmering soup. Cook and stir until slightly thickened and the starchy taste is gone.

Diced cooked chicken or
   turkey with the fat and skin
   removed . . . . .3 pounds,
                4 ounces
                (about 2 1/2
                quarts)
Precooked rice . . . . .2 quarts
			4. Add chicken or turkey and rice to soup. Stir to mix well. Reheat to serving temperature, if necessary, and serve hot.

Potato Soup

Refer to footnotes for special dietary information

INGREDIENTS WEIGHTS/MEASURES	YIELD ADJUST.	METHOD
Diced fresh white potatoes. . . .3 quarts Boiling water. . . . . .5 quarts Salt . . . . .3 tablespoons Milk . . . . .as necessary		1. Cook potatoes with water and salt over medium heat until potatoes are tender. 2. Drain potatoes; save potato water; add enough milk to potato water to total 2 gallons.
Finely chopped onions. . . . . . .1 cup Margarine . . . . .1 cup (8 ounces)		3. Fry onions in margarine, over low heat, 10 minutes, stirring occasionally.
All-purpose flour . . . . .3/4 cup White pepper. . . . . .1 teaspoon		4. Stir flour and pepper into onions and fat; cook and stir over low heat until smooth; add flour mixture to lukewarm milk and potato water; cook, stirring constantly, over moderate heat until smooth and thickened and the starchy taste is gone. 5. Add potatoes to hot soup; heat to serving temperature; serve hot.

YIELD
50 portions (about 2½ gallons)

PORTION SIZE
¾ cup (6-ounce ladle)

PAN SIZE
Heavy 5-gallon pot

DIETARY INFORMATION
May be used as written for general, no added salt and mechanical soft diets. Diabetic diets — each serving provides 1 skim milk and 1 fat exchanges. Bland diets — omit pepper. Low cholesterol diets — use skim milk in step 2.

YIELD
50 portions (about 2½ gallons)

PORTION SIZE
¾ cup (6-ounce ladle)

PAN SIZE
Heavy 5-gallon pot

DIETARY INFORMATION
May be used as written for general and no added salt diets. Diabetic diets — each serving provides 1 vegetable, 1 lean meat and 1 fat exchanges. Bland diets — omit pepper and fresh peppers. Low cholesterol diets — use margarine in step 2. Each serving provides 1 ounce fish.

Salmon Chowder

Refer to footnotes for special dietary information

INGREDIENTS	WEIGHTS/MEASURES	YIELD ADJUST.	METHOD
Canned salmon	4 1-pound cans		1. Drain salmon; save juice for use in step 3; discard skin and bones; break salmon into smaller pieces.
Chopped onions Chopped fresh green peppers Margarine or bacon fat	1½ quarts 1 quart ¾ cup		2. Fry onions and green peppers in margarine or bacon fat in pot until onions are golden.
Crushed canned tomatoes and juice Chicken broth Chopped drained canned green beans Canned drained whole kernel corn Salt Pepper Ground thyme	2 quarts (⅔ No. 10 can) 1 gallon 1½ quarts (½ No. 10 can) 1 quart (⅓ No. 10 can) 1 tablespoon 1 teaspoon 2 teaspoons		3. Add salmon juice, tomatoes, broth, beans, corn, salt, pepper and thyme to onions; simmer 15 minutes.
Instant potatoes	3 cups		4. Stir potatoes into chowder; simmer another 5 minutes.
Lemon juice	¼ cup		5. Add lemon juice and salmon pieces to chowder; heat to serving temperature; serve hot.

Split Pea Soup

Refer to footnotes for special dietary information

INGREDIENTS	WEIGHTS/MEASURES	YIELD ADJUST.	METHOD
Dry split peas	3 pounds, 8 ounces (2 quarts)		1. Pick over peas; remove any foreign matter; wash thoroughly in cold water.
Cold water	1½ gallons		2. Cover peas with the 1½ gallons cold water; bring to a boil; cook 2 minutes; turn off heat; let stand 1 hour.
Finely diced bacon	1 pound, 4 ounces		3. Fry bacon until crisp; remove bacon from fat with a slotted spoon; add bacon to split peas; keep bacon fat for use in step 5.
Ham stock or water	1¼ gallons		4. Add stock or water, onions, carrots, celery salt and bay leaves to split peas; simmer 1 hour or until peas are mushy.
Finely chopped onions	2 cups		
Grated carrots	1¼ cups		
Celery salt	1½ tablespoons		
Bay leaves	2 each		
All-purpose flour	⅓ cup		5. Stir flour into bacon fat; stir until smooth; add to soup; cook and stir until thickened; add ham and simmer another 10 minutes, stirring frequently. Add salt and pepper to soup, if necessary, and serve hot.
Diced cooked ham	1 pound		
Salt and pepper	as necessary		

YIELD
50 portions (about 2½ gallons)

PORTION SIZE
¾ cup (6-ounce ladle)

PAN SIZE
Heavy 5-gallon pot

DIETARY INFORMATION
May be used as written for general, no added salt and mechanical soft diets. Diabetic diets — each serving provides 1 bread, 1 vegetable, 1 lean meat and 1 fat exchanges. Bland diets — omit pepper. Each serving provides 1 ounce meat and equivalent.

YIELD
50 portions (about 2½ gallons)

PORTION SIZE
¾ cup (6-ounce ladle)

PAN SIZE
Heavy 5-gallon pot

NOTE
If desired, beef stock may be prepared from beef soup base using the amount specified on the container for 1¾ gallons stock and 3 pounds, 2 ounces of diced precooked beef may be substituted for the beef stew meat and water in steps 1 and 2.

DIETARY INFORMATION
May be used as written for general, no added salt and mechanical soft diets. Diabetic diets — each serving provides 1 lean meat and 1 vegetable exchanges. Bland diets — omit pepper. Each serving provides 1 ounce beef.

Vegetable Beef Soup

Refer to footnotes for special dietary information

INGREDIENTS	WEIGHTS/MEASURES	YIELD ADJUST.	METHOD
Boneless beef stew meat, cut in ½-inch cubes .... 5 pounds Cold water................. 2 gallons Salt .... 2 tablespoons Bay leaves................. 2 Pepper.................... 1 teaspoon Cold water................. as necessary			1. Put stew meat, 2 gallons water, salt, bay leaves and pepper in pot; simmer 1 to 1½ hours or until meat is tender. Drain stock from meat; refrigerate meat; put stock in refrigerator; chill until fat rises to the top; discard fat. 2. Measure stock after fat has been discarded. If there is less than 1¾ gallons stock, add enough water to total 1¾ gallons; return stock to heat.
Chopped parsley............ ¼ cup Diced fresh white potatoes.... 1½ quarts Diced celery .... 1 cup Diced carrots .... 3 cups Chopped onions .... 3 cups Shredded cabbage .... 3 cups Canned drained crushed tomatoes (optional)........ 1 quart (⅓ No. 10 can)			3. Add parsley, potatoes, celery, carrots, onions, cabbage and tomatoes to beef stock; simmer 30 minutes.
Salt .... 2 tablespoons			4. Add salt, and cooked meat to soup, simmer another 5 minutes. Serve hot.

Salt Free Chicken or Beef Broth

Refer to footnotes for special dietary information

INGREDIENTS	WEIGHTS/MEASURES	YIELD ADJUST.	METHOD
Chicken necks and backs.....15 pounds or cut beef bones ....15 pounds			1. Place chicken necks and backs in pot. Rinse thoroughly 2 or 3 times and drain well. Or place beef bones in large roasting pan and roast, uncovered, until well browned. (This browning step is very important for a full-bodied, flavorful stock.) Discard fat and place browned bones in pot.
Cool water................6 gallons Coarsely chopped carrots ....1½ cups Coarsely chopped onions.....1½ cups Coarsely chopped celery .....1½ cups Bay leaves................2 Thyme...................1 teaspoon			2. Pour water over bones. Cover and bring to a simmer. Add carrots, onions, celery, bay leaves and thyme. Cover and simmer 3 or 4 hours or until chicken and/or meat is falling off the bones. 3. Strain broth off meat into a clean container using a strainer or china cap.
Yellow food coloring ....as necessary Caramel food coloring ....as necessary			4. Add yellow food coloring to chicken broth or caramel coloring to beef broth, if necessary. Set the pot in a sink with cold water in it and cool the broth, stirring it occasionally, until the broth is lukewarm. Refrigerate until needed. 5. Skim any fat off the top of the broth and use as desired.

YIELD
5 to 6 gallons

PORTION SIZE
As needed

PAN SIZE
Heavy 10-gallon pot

TEMPERATURE
375°F. Oven

DIETARY INFORMATION
May be used as desired for general, no added salt, bland, soft, mechanical soft, restricted residue, low fat and low cholesterol diets. Diabetic diets — this recipe may be considered free as written.

Chapter 4
Meats

Meat Information

Meat, poultry and fish account for a big percentage of food expenditures and it is a wise administrator who manages to get the most food for his dollar. Very few administrators are trained buyers but there are a few points which it is well for all buyers to observe.

1. A good supplier is very important. The buyer should try to have a supplier who will discuss the problems of the buyer. A good supplier can help the buyer know what is available, what is in long supply and therefore a little more reasonable and what new items are available on the market.

2. Food should be bought according to specification. The specifications can be formal written agreements or they can be a simple set of instructions from the buyer to the supplier. The buyer and supplier should spend time together to be sure that both of them understand what the buyer needs and wants. The recipes in this book indicate the cuts of meat, fish and poultry needed for each recipe and can be useful in determining the specifications for those items. The supplier needs to know the exact size pork chops and other portion cut meats, the size of stew meat and the cut it is fabricated from and whether cube steaks should go through the machine once or twice. It is particularly important that they understand each other regarding the amount of fat in ground beef. This will vary from a high of 30% for regular hamburger to a low of about 15% for ground round. Generally speaking, lean beef with 20% fat will yield a satisfactory beef patty without too much cooking loss.

3. The cost per serving of meat, fish and poultry is more important than the cost per pound. A pound of 4-ounce veal cutlets will serve 4 people and it is a good buy if it is less than twice the cost of short ribs of beef which would only serve 2 people.

4. A good heavy-duty scale should be purchased and all of the meat which comes into the kitchen should be weighed. The weight of the meat should be checked before the delivery ticket is signed. Even the most reputable supplier will occasionally make mistakes and it is hard to check the mistakes without an accurate scale.

5. After meat is purchased, it should be cooked according to the recipe. Cooks should be instructed to follow the recipes very closely and be sure the ovens are registering the correct temperatures. Most cooks do not realize that 10 to 15% more weight can be lost from a roast which is cooked at 375°F. instead of at 325°F. It should be stressed that each 3 ounces of meat which is lost because the meat is cooked at a higher temperature means that a serving of roast is lost and the food cost will be higher for all of the remaining servings.

Good or choice meats are generally considered the best buy for institutions. Prime meat is generally quite expensive, and lower grades are often too difficult to cook to be as tender as necessary. Therefore, most buyers agree that good or choice grade is most satisfactory on all points.

6. The storage of fresh and cooked meat is as important as the correct storage of frozen meat. The following principles should be used in the storage of meat.

a. Fresh meat should be stored in the coldest part of the refrigerator. The temperature should be as low as possible without freezing the meat (about 38°F.).

b. Pre-packaged fresh meat may be stored in the refrigerator in the original wrapping for not over 2 days. It may be stored in the freezer without rewrapping for 1 to 2 weeks. It must be rewrapped in special freezer paper if it is to be stored longer than 1 or 2 weeks.

c. Fresh meat which was not pre-packaged should be removed from the wrapping paper and wrapped loosely in wax paper or aluminum foil. It may be refrigerated for up to 2 days.

d. Variety meats and ground or chopped meats are more perishable than other meats and should be cooked in 1 to 2 days if not frozen.

e. Cured, cured and smoked meat and sausages should be stored in the refrigerator. They should be left in their original wrappings. Canned hams and other perishable canned meats should be stored in the refrigerator unless storage recommendations on the can state otherwise. These meats should not be frozen.

f. Frozen meat should be put in the freezer as soon as it is delivered unless it is to be defrosted for cooking. It is a good idea to date the packages as they are put in the freezer as a guide to their age. Storage time should be limited in order to use them at their best flavor and palatability. The temperature of the freezer should be kept at 0°F. or colder.

g. Leftover cooked meat should be cooled as rapidly as possible, then covered or wrapped and stored in the refrigerator. Creamed dishes should be cooled to lukewarm by putting the container in a sink surrounded by cold water. Roasts should be allowed to stand at room temperature for a few minutes and then be put into the refrigerator. It is not necessary to cool meats to room temperatures before they are put into the refrigerator.

h. Leftover meat should be left in as big pieces as possible to prevent bacterial contamination. Bones may be removed to save space, if necessary, but meat should not be chopped, sliced or ground until it is to be used.

7. Frozen meat may be defrosted before it is cooked or it may be cooked from the frozen state, if necessary. It is important to allow additional cooking times for meats which are to be cooked from the frozen state. Frozen roasts require about an additional 30 to 50% cooking time depending upon the thickness of the meat. Additional cooking time for steaks and chops will vary according to the thickness of the meat.

The most desirable method for defrosting frozen meat is in the refrigerator. The meat should be defrosted in its original wrapping. Defrosting in water is not recommended unless the meat is to be cooked in the liquid.

After meat is defrosted, it should be cooked in the same way as fresh meat which has not been frozen. A roast will generally take 3 to 7 hours to defrost depending upon the size of the roast.

It is not a good idea to refreeze meat which has been defrosted because of the danger of contamination while it was being defrosted.

THE MEAT BUYERS' GUIDE, published by the National Association of Meat Purveyors, 8365 Greensboro Drive, McLean, Virginia 22102 can be used for detailed descriptions of different meat cuts and how to buy them. It includes pictures and descriptions of standardized cuts and can be very helpful to new or inexperienced cooks and buyers.

YIELD
50 portions

PORTION SIZE
3 ounces

PAN SIZE
18 × 24-inch roasting pan

TEMPERATURE
325°F. Oven

NOTE
If frozen meats are used, they should be cooked 3 to 3½ hours.

DIETARY INFORMATION
May be used as written for general and no added salt diets. Diabetic diets — each serving provides 3 lean meat exchanges. Bland and restricted residue diets — omit pepper. Low fat and low cholesterol diets — remove all visible fat and do not serve with gravy. Each serving provides 3 ounces cooked beef.

Roast Beef

Refer to footnotes for special dietary information

INGREDIENTS	WEIGHTS/MEASURES	YIELD ADJUST.	METHOD
Boneless beef roast (rump, sirloin, rolled roast, 4 to 6 pounds)................	14 pounds, 8 ounces		1. Rub each roast with salt and pepper. 2. Place roasts, fat side up, in pan without crowding; do not cover pan or add water. 3. Insert meat thermometer in thickest part of meat; cook to an internal temperature of 140°F. (rare), 160°F. (medium) or 170°F. (well). Or cook in oven 2 to 2½ hours depending upon size of roast. 4. Remove meat from pan; cool 20 to 30 minutes before slicing. (If meat is not to be used immediately, it should be refrigerated after 30 minutes.) 5. Use any drippings for making gravy. If gravy is not to be made immediately, drippings should be refrigerated until used. (Scrape brown particles from pan and store with drippings for gravy.)
Salt	1½ tablespoons		
Pepper	1½ teaspoons		

Beef Pot Roast

Refer to footnotes for special dietary information

INGREDIENTS	WEIGHTS/MEASURES	YIELD ADJUST.	METHOD
Boneless beef roast (rolled chuck, pot roast or rump) . . .14 pounds, 8 ounces			1. Put roasts in pan without crowding; sprinkle with salt and pepper; scatter carrots and onions over roasts; pour hot water in bottom of pan; cover tightly.
Salt .1½ tablespoons			2. Cook meat in oven 3 to 4 hours or until tender; turn roasts 2 or 3 times during cooking period; add a small amount of hot water, if necessary.
Pepper. . . . . .1½ teaspoons			3. Remove meat from pan; cool 20 to 30 minutes before slicing. (If meat is not to be used immediately, it should be refrigerated after 30 minutes.)
Chopped carrots. . . . . .1 cup			
Chopped onions . . . . .1 cup			
Hot water . . . . .2 cups			4. Skim as much fat as possible off drippings and use for making gravy. If gravy is not to be made immediately, drippings should be refrigerated until used. Fat should be removed from top of drippings, if they have been refrigerated, before they are used. Brown particles should be scraped from pan and stored with drippings for gravy. A little boiling hot water can be used to wash brown particles out of the pan for storage.

YIELD
50 portions

PORTION SIZE
3 ounces

PAN SIZE
Roasting pan

TEMPERATURE
325°F. Oven

VARIATION
1. Hot beef sandwich: Put 3 ounces of thinly sliced beef between 2 slices of bread; pour ⅓ cup hot brown gravy over sandwich.

NOTES
1. If frozen roasts are used, they should be cooked 4 to 5 hours. 2. This amount of roast will yield 75 2-ounce portions of beef for hot beef sandwiches.

DIETARY INFORMATION
May be used as written for general and no added salt diets. Diabetic diets — each serving provides 3 lean meat exchanges. Bland and restricted residue diets — omit pepper. Low cholesterol and low fat diets — remove all visible fat and do not serve with gravy. Each serving provides 3 ounces cooked beef.

YIELD
50 portions

PORTION SIZE
3 ounces

PAN SIZE
Heavy 5-gallon pot

DIETARY INFORMATION
May be used as written for general, bland and no added salt diets. Diabetic diets — each serving provides 3 lean meat exchanges. Low cholesterol and low fat diets — remove all visible fat. Each serving provides 3 ounces cooked corned beef.

Corned Beef

Refer to footnotes for special dietary information

INGREDIENTS	WEIGHTS/MEASURES	YIELD ADJUST.	METHOD
Boneless corned brisket of beef	15 pounds, 12 ounces		1. Put whole pieces of beef in heavy pot; cover with cold water; bring to a boil; cover; reduce heat and simmer 4 to 5 hours depending upon size of the pieces. Test each piece with a fork after 4 hours and remove any tender pieces; continue to simmer until all pieces are tender.
Cold water	as necessary		2. Remove any scum which comes to the surface while corned beef is cooking.
			3. When all pieces are tender, remove from range and add pieces which were taken out of the liquid earlier; let stand 20 minutes; remove pieces from liquid to a pan and let stand 20 minutes before slicing. (If meat is not to be served immediately, it should be refrigerated now.)
			4. Slice across grain when serving corned beef. The meat will have to be turned in several directions while it is being sliced because the grain of the brisket runs in many directions.

Braised Short Ribs of Beef

Refer to footnotes for special dietary information

INGREDIENTS	WEIGHTS/MEASURES	YIELD ADJUST.	METHOD
Short ribs of beef . . . . .25 pounds (50 8-oz. portions) Salt . . . . .¼ cup Pepper . . . . .1 teaspoon All-purpose flour . . . . .3 cups Paprika . . . . .3 tablespoons Hot water . . . . .1 quart			1. Combine salt, pepper, flour and paprika; mix well. 2. Dip short ribs in flour mixture; put ribs in a single layer on lightly greased sheet pans; bake at 450°F. for 45 minutes; pour off fat and put short ribs in a roasting pan; use hot water to scrape the brown bits from the pan; add hot water and brown bits to roasting pan with the short ribs.
Tomato puree . . . . .2 cups Salt . . . . .1 tablespoon Finely chopped onions . . . . . . .2 cups Finely chopped carrots. . . . . . .2 cups Finely chopped celery . . . . . . .1 cup			3. Add tomato puree, salt, onions, carrots and celery to short ribs; cover pan and bake at 350°F. for about 2 hours or until very tender. 4. Remove roaster from oven to top of range; put short ribs in steam table pans and skim excess fat from sauce.
All-purpose flour . . . . .1 cup Cold water. . . . . .2 cups Hot water . . . . .2 quarts Cold water. . . . . .as necessary			5. Stir flour and 2 cups cold water together to form a smooth paste; add hot water to drippings in pan and stir to mix well; add flour mixture to gravy and cook and stir until smooth and thickened. Add more cold water to the gravy if it is too thick; cook and stir until well blended and the starchy taste is gone.

YIELD
50 portions

PORTION SIZE
1 piece plus gravy

PAN SIZE
18 × 26-inch sheet pans
Roasting pan

TEMPERATURE
450°F. and 350°F. Oven

DIETARY INFORMATION
May be used as written for general and no added salt diets. Diabetic diets — each serving, without gravy, provides 3 lean meat and 2 vegetable exchanges. Bland diets — omit pepper. Each serving provides 3 ounces cooked beef.

YIELD
50 portions (2 pans)

PORTION SIZE
1 steak plus ¼ cup (2-ounce ladle) gravy

PAN SIZE
18 × 26-inch sheet pans

TEMPERATURE
375°F. and 325°F. Oven

DIETARY INFORMATION
May be used as written for general and no added salt diets. Bland diets — omit pepper. Each serving provides 3 ounces cooked beef.

Baked Cube Steak

Refer to footnotes for special dietary information

INGREDIENTS	WEIGHTS/MEASURES	YIELD ADJUST.	METHOD
All-purpose flour . . . . .2 quarts Onion salt . . . . .2 teaspoons Paprika . . . . .3 tablespoons Pepper. . . . . .½ teaspoon Salt . . . . .2 tablespoons			1. Sift flour, onion salt, paprika, pepper, and salt together into a shallow pan; mix well. (The amount of this mixture used will depend upon the size of the steaks.)
Vegetable oil . . . . .as necessary Cubed beef steaks . . . . .12 pounds, 8 ounces (50 4-oz. steaks)			2. Pour oil in shallow pan; dip steaks in oil; drain well in a colander. 3. Dredge drained steaks in flour mixture; put on well-greased sheet pans and bake at 375°F. for 20 minutes; reduce heat and bake at 325°F. until tender but not more than 20 minutes. The length of time will depend upon the tenderness of the meat.

Fiesta Baked Steak

Refer to footnotes for special dietary information

INGREDIENTS	WEIGHTS/MEASURES	YIELD ADJUST.	METHOD
All-purpose flour . . . . .2 cups Salt . . . . .¼ cup Pepper . . . . .2 teaspoons			1. Combine flour, salt and pepper; mix well.
Cubed beef steaks . . . . .12 pounds, 8 ounces (50 4-oz. steaks)			2. Dredge steaks in seasoned flour; save any excess flour for use in step 4.
Vegetable oil . . . . .1 cup			3. Heat ½ of the vegetable oil in each of 2 sheet pans; arrange 25 floured steaks in each pan; bake 10 minutes; turn over and continue to bake another 10 minutes; arrange 25 steaks, shingle style, in each of 2 greased steam table pans.
Crushed canned tomatoes . . . .1½ quarts (½ No. 10 can) Oregano . . . . .1½ tablespoons			4. Combine remaining flour with ½ cup of the juice of the tomatoes; mix until smooth; add to tomatoes along with oregano and mix well.
Onions, sliced about ¼-inch thick . . . . .6 large sweet onions Paprika . . . . .1½ tablespoons			5. Arrange half of the onion rings over each pan of meat; pour half of the tomato sauce over each pan of meat and onion rings; sprinkle with paprika. 6. Cover tightly with aluminum foil and bake 1 hour or until tender.

YIELD
50 portions (2 pans)

PORTION SIZE
1 steak plus sauce

PAN SIZE
18 × 26-inch sheet pans
12 × 20 × 2-inch steam table pans

TEMPERATURE
375°F. Oven

NOTES
Portion cut beef steak (4 ounces, cut ¾-inch thick) may be used instead of cube steak. Bake meat 30 minutes on each side in step 3 and bake 1½ hours or until tender in step 6.

DIETARY INFORMATION
May be used as written for general, no added salt, and low cholesterol diets. Diabetic diets — each serving provides 3½ lean meat and 1 vegetable exchanges. Bland diets — omit pepper. Each serving provides 3 ounces of cooked beef.

YIELD
50 portions (2 pans)

PORTION SIZE
1 steak plus sauce

PAN SIZE
18 × 26-inch sheet pans
Heavy 3-gallon pot
12 × 20 × 2-inch steam table pans

TEMPERATURE
375°F. and 325°F. Oven

VARIATION
Swiss steak with brown gravy: Use 1 gallon hot beef stock instead of soup and water in step 5.

NOTE
Portion cut beef steak (4 ounces, cut 3/4-inch thick) may be used instead of cube steak; brown meat 20 minutes on each side in step 3 and cook about 1 1/2 hours or until tender in step 6.

DIETARY INFORMATION
May be used as written for general and no added salt diets. Diabetic diets — each serving provides 3 lean meat and 2 vegetable exchanges. Bland diets — omit pepper. Each serving provides 3 ounces cooked beef.

Swiss Steak with Tomato Sauce

Refer to footnotes for special dietary information

INGREDIENTS	WEIGHTS/MEASURES	YIELD ADJUST.	METHOD
All-purpose flour . . . . .2 cups Salt .1/4 cup Pepper . . . . .2 teaspoons			1. Combine flour, salt and pepper and mix well.
Cubed beef steaks . . . . .12 pounds, 8 ounces (50 4-ounce steaks)			2. Dredge steaks in seasoned flour.
Vegetable oil . . . . .1/2 cup			3. Heat 1/2 of the oil in each of 2 sheet pans; arrange 25 floured steaks in each pan; bake in the oven at 375°F. for 10 minutes; turn over and continue to bake for another 10 minutes; arrange 25 steaks, shingle style, in each of 2 greased steam table pans.
Finely chopped onions . . . . . . .1 quart Finely chopped celery . . . . . . .1 quart Shortening . . . . .1/4 cup			4. Fry onions and celery in shortening in pot until onions are golden.
Condensed cream of tomato soup . . . . .2 46-ounce cans (3 quarts) Hot water . . . . .3 quarts			5. Add soup and water to hot vegetables; mix well; heat to a simmer; pour half of the mixture over meat in each pan; cover tightly with aluminum foil. 6. Bake at 325°F. for 45 minutes; uncover pans and continue to bake another 30 minutes or until steaks are tender.

Baked Beef and Noodles

Refer to footnotes for special dietary information

INGREDIENTS / WEIGHTS/MEASURES	YIELD ADJUST.	METHOD
Diced boneless beef . . . . .14 pounds Chopped onions . . . . .2 cups Salt . . . . .1 tablespoon		1. Put beef in roasting pan; do not add any shortening; sprinkle onions and salt over meat and cook, uncovered, about 1 hour or until meat is browned; drain off as much fat as possible.
Hot water . . . . .2 quarts		2. Pour hot water over meat; cover and and bake 1½ to 2 hours or until the meat is tender.
Noodles. . . . . .3 pounds Boiling water. . . . . .3 gallons Salt . . . . .3 tablespoons Vegetable oil . . . . .2 tablespoons		3. Stir noodles into boiling salted water; add vegetable oil and cook, stirring occasionally, 12 to 15 minutes or until tender; drain well.
Shortening, melted . . . . .½ cup All-purpose flour . . . . .2 cups Hot beef stock . . . . .1¼ gallons		4. Mix shortening and flour together until smooth; add to hot stock; cook and stir over moderate heat for 10 minutes or until smooth and thickened.
Tomato catsup . . . . .1 cup Salt . . . . .3 tablespoons Pepper. . . . . .1 teaspoon		5. Add catsup, salt and pepper to hot sauce (the amount of salt will vary depending upon saltiness of the beef stock in step 4); mix well; add noodles and beef to sauce; mix well and pour into greased roasting pan.
Dry bread crumbs . . . . .1 cup (4 ounces)		6. Sprinkle bread crumbs over noodle mixture and bake 1 hour.

YIELD
50 portions

PORTION SIZE
1 cup (8 ounces)

PAN SIZE
Heavy 5-gallon pot
Roasting pan

TEMPERATURE
350°F. Oven

DIETARY INFORMATION
May be used as written for general and no salt added diets. Diabetic diets — each serving provides 4 lean meat and 1½ bread exchanges. Bland diets — omit pepper. Each serving provides 3 ounces cooked beef.

YIELD
50 portions (about 2 gallons)

PORTION SIZE
5 ounces

PAN SIZE
Roasting pan

TEMPERATURE
350°F. Oven

DIETARY INFORMATION
May be used as written for general, bland and no added salt diets. Diabetic diets — each serving provides 3 lean meat and 1 vegetable exchanges. Each serving provides 3 ounces cooked beef.

Beef Cubes with Sour Cream

Refer to footnotes for special dietary information

INGREDIENTS	WEIGHTS/MEASURES	YIELD ADJUST.	METHOD
Diced boneless beef . . . . .14 pounds Chopped onions . . . . .1 quart Salt . . . . .2 tablespoons			1. Put beef in roasting pan; do not add any shortening; sprinkle onions and salt over meat and roast, uncovered, about 1 hour or until meat is browned; drain off as much fat as possible.
Hot water . . . . .2½ quarts			2. Pour hot water over meat; cover and bake about 1½ to 2 hours or until meat is tender; put roaster on top of range; drain off as much fat as possible from drippings; return drippings to meat.
Canned mushrooms . . . . .2 1-pound cans			3. Drain mushrooms; keep juice for use in step 4; add mushrooms to meat.
All-purpose flour . . . . .1 cup Mushroom juice plus cold water . . . . .2 cups			4. Stir flour into mushroom juice and water to form a smooth paste; stir into meat gradually; cook and stir over moderate heat until smooth and thickened and the starchy taste is gone; remove from heat.
Sour cream (room temperature) . . . . . . .2 quarts			5. Stir sour cream carefully into meat and gravy; reheat but DO NOT BOIL; serve hot.

Beef Medley

Refer to footnotes for special dietary information

INGREDIENTS	WEIGHTS/MEASURES	YIELD ADJUST.	METHOD
Diced boneless beef . . . . 14 pounds Salt . . . . ¼ cup			1. Put beef in roasting pan; do not add any shortening; sprinkle salt over meat and roast, uncovered, about 1 hour or until meat is browned; drain off as much fat as possible.
Hot water . . . . .2 quarts			2. Pour hot water over meat; cover tightly and bake about 1 to 1½ hours or until meat is tender; put meat in a colander and drain well; put ½ of the meat in each of 2 steam table pans; remove as much fat as possible from drippings and then put half of the drippings in each steam table pan with the meat.
Finely chopped onions . . . . . . .1 cup Chopped fresh green peppers .2 cups Chopped fresh parsley . . . . . . .½ cup Vegetable oil . . . . .¼ cup			3. Fry onions, fresh green peppers and parsley in oil until onions are golden; put ½ of the fried vegetables in each of the pans.
Chopped pimiento . . . . .½ cup Uncooked rice. . . . . .3 pounds, 8 ounces (2 quarts) Hot beef stock . . . . .2 quarts Tomato juice . . . . .1½ quarts Ground oregano . . . . .1 tablespoon Salt . . . . .2 tablespoons Pepper. . . . . .1½ teaspoons			4. Put ½ of the pimiento, rice, beef stock, tomato juice, oregano, salt and pepper into each of the 2 pans with the meat; mix each pan lightly but well; cover tightly with aluminum foil and bake 45 minutes or until rice is tender.

YIELD
50 portions (2 pans)

PORTION SIZE
¾ cup (6 ounces)

PAN SIZE
Roasting pan
12 × 20 × 2-inch steam table pans

TEMPERATURE
325°F. Oven

DIETARY INFORMATION
May be used as written for general and no added salt diets. Diabetic diets — each serving provides 4 lean meat and 1½ bread exchanges. Bland diets — omit fresh green peppers and pepper. Low cholesterol diets — remove all visible fat from meat before it is cooked. Each serving provides 3 ounces cooked beef.

YIELD
50 portions (about 3¼ gallons)

PORTION SIZE
1 cup (8 ounces)

PAN SIZE
Roasting pan
Heavy 3-gallon pot

TEMPERATURE
375°F. Oven

NOTE
Rotini is a screw shaped macaroni. If it is not available, shell or elbow macaroni may be substituted and cooked only 5 minutes in step 3.

DIETARY INFORMATION
May be used as written for general and no added salt diets. Diabetic diets — each serving provides 4 lean meat and 1½ bread exchanges. Bland diets — omit pepper. Low cholesterol diets — remove all visible fat from meat before it is cooked. Each serving provides 3 ounces cooked beef.

Beef Rotini

Refer to footnotes for special dietary information

INGREDIENTS	WEIGHTS/MEASURES	YIELD ADJUST.	METHOD
Diced boneless beef . . . . .14 pounds Chopped onions . . . . .1 quart Salt . . . . .2 tablespoons			1. Put meat in roasting pan; do not add any shortening; sprinkle onions and salt over meat and roast, uncovered, about 1 hour or until meat is browned; drain off as much fat as possible.
Hot water . . . . .2 quarts			2. Pour hot water over meat; cover tightly and continue to bake 1 to 1½ hours or until tender; drain off as much fat as possible.
Rotini. . . . . .2 pounds Hot water . . . . .2 gallons Salt . . . . .2 tablespoons Vegetable oil . . . . .2 tablespoons			3. Drop rotini into boiling salted water; stir lightly to mix; add oil and cook, uncovered, 10 minutes; drain (the rotini will not be tender yet.)
Tomato sauce . . . . .2 quarts Pepper . . . . .1 teaspoon			4. Stir tomato sauce and pepper in with meat; add hot drained rotini and mix well; cover tightly and continue to bake another 30 minutes or until rotini is tender.
Hot drained canned peas . . . . .3 quarts (1 No. 10 can) Grated Parmesan cheese . . . . .about 1 cup			5. Fold peas into meat mixture and serve hot; sprinkle about 1 teaspoon cheese on top of each serving.

Beef Stew

Refer to footnotes for special dietary information

INGREDIENTS	WEIGHTS/MEASURES	YIELD ADJUST.	METHOD
Diced boneless beef . . . . 14 pounds Chopped onions . . . . 2 cups Salt . . . . ¼ cup			1. Put meat in roasting pan; do not add any shortening; sprinkle onions and salt over meat and roast, uncovered, about 1 hour or until meat is browned; drain off as much fat as possible.
Hot water . . . . 1 gallon			2. Pour hot water over meat; cover tightly and continue to bake 1 to 1½ hours or until tender; drain off as much fat as possible from drippings; return drippings to meat; remove cover and put roaster on top of the range.
Carrots, cut in 1-inch pieces . . . 3 quarts Celery, cut in 1-inch pieces . . . . 2 quarts Potatoes, cut in 1-inch cubes . . 2½ quarts Salt . . . . 2 tablespoons Hot water . . . . to cover			3. Cover vegetables with hot water; add salt; bring to a boil; cover and cook about 20 minutes or until vegetables are tender; drain vegetables well but save the liquid to use for gravy, if necessary.
All-purpose flour . . . . 2 cups Cold water . . . . 1 quart			4. Combine flour and water and mix until smooth; add to meat and juice; cook and stir over medium heat until thickened and smooth and the starchy taste is gone; add as much vegetable liquid as necessary for a medium thick gravy.
Drained canned peas . . . . 3 quarts (1 No. 10 can)			5. Add peas and vegetables to meat and gravy; add salt, if necessary; mix lightly; serve hot.

YIELD
50 portions (about 3¼ gallons)

PORTION SIZE
1 cup (8-ounce ladle)

PAN SIZE
Roasting pan
Heavy 3-gallon pot

TEMPERATURE
350°F. Oven

NOTE
3 No. 10 cans of drained, canned mixed vegetables may be used instead of the carrots, celery, potatoes and peas. Heat vegetables in their own liquid before adding them to the stew; drain well and use the liquid from the canned vegetables to thin the gravy, if necessary, in step 5.

DIETARY INFORMATION
May be used as written for general, bland and no added salt diets. Diabetic diets — each serving provides 3 lean meat and 3 vegetable exchanges. Low cholesterol diets — remove all visible fat from meat before it is cooked. Each serving provides 3 ounces cooked beef.

Baked Hamburgers

Refer to footnotes for special dietary information

YIELD
50 portions

PORTION SIZE
1 hamburger patty

PAN SIZE
18 × 26-inch sheet pans

TEMPERATURE
400°F. Oven

VARIATIONS
1. Beefburgers: Combine 13 pounds lean ground beef with 2 tablespoons salt and 2 cups ice water; mix, shape and bake as directed in basic recipe.
2. Broiled hamburgers: Mix and shape patties according to steps 1 and 2 in basic recipe. Broil hamburgers about 4 inches from heat about 5 to 6 minutes on each side.

DIETARY INFORMATION
May be used as written for general, no added salt, bland (omit pepper) and mechanical soft diets. Diabetic diets — each serving provides 3 lean meat and ½ vegetable exchanges. Bland diets — omit pepper. Restricted residue diets — omit onions and pepper. Each serving provides 3 ounces cooked beef.

INGREDIENTS	WEIGHTS/MEASURES	YIELD ADJUST.	METHOD
Lean ground beef . . . . .13 pounds Dry bread crumbs . . . . .2 cups Finely chopped onions . . . . . . .1 cup Salt . . . . .2 tablespoons Pepper. . . . . .½ teaspoon Slightly beaten eggs . . . . .½ cup (2 to 3 medium) Cool water. . . . . .2 cups			1. Put all ingredients in mixer bowl in order listed; mix at low speed for 2 to 4 minutes or until well blended; DO NOT OVERMIX. 2. Use a No. 12 dipper to shape the meat into 4-ounce rounds; flatten rounds to about 4 inches in diameter. Weigh several patties to check their weight. 3. Bake 15 to 20 minutes or until the center is no longer pink.

Beefaroni

Refer to footnotes for special dietary information

INGREDIENTS	WEIGHTS/MEASURES	YIELD ADJUST.	METHOD
Chopped onions . . . . .2 quarts Chopped fresh green peppers .2 quarts Vegetable oil . . . . .¼ cup Ground beef . . . . .8 pounds, 12 ounces			1. Fry onions and green peppers in oil until onions are golden; add beef; cook and stir until meat is well browned; pour meat into a colander; drain off fat; discard fat and return meat to heat.
Tomato puree . . . . .3 quarts (1 No. 10 can) Beef soup base . . . . .½ cup Worcestershire sauce . . . . . . .½ cup Ground oregano . . . . .1 tablespoon Basil . . . . .1 teaspoon Ground cloves . . . . .¼ teaspoon Garlic powder . . . . .1 teaspoon Salt . . . . .2 tablespoons Pepper . . . . .1 teaspoon Hot water . . . . .1 gallon			2. Add tomato puree, soup base, Worcestershire sauce, oregano, basil, cloves, garlic, salt, pepper and hot water to meat; bring to a boil; reduce heat and simmer, covered, 30 minutes, stirring occasionally.
Elbow macaroni . . . . .2 pounds, 8 ounces			3. Add macaroni to meat mixture; bring to a boil; reduce heat and simmer, covered, about 20 minutes or until macaroni is tender; add more water and salt, if necessary. Serve hot.

YIELD
50 portions (about 3¼ gallons)

PORTION SIZE
1 cup (8-ounce ladle)

PAN SIZE
Heavy 5-gallon pot

DIETARY INFORMATION
May be used as written for general, no added salt, low cholesterol and mechanical soft diets. Diabetic diets — each serving provides 2 lean meat, 1 bread and 2 vegetable exchanges. Bland diet — omit fresh green peppers and pepper. Each serving provides 2 ounces cooked beef.

YIELD
50 portions (2 pans)

PORTION SIZE
1 cup (8 ounces)

PAN SIZE
Heavy 5-gallon pot
12 × 20 × 2-inch steam table pans

TEMPERATURE
350°F. Oven

NOTE
1. Beef and noodles may be served hot without baking, if desired.
2. 13 pounds ground beef may be substituted for 8 pounds 12 ounces ground beef in step 2, and noodles decreased to 3 pounds in step 1 to yield 50 1-cup portions providing 3 ounces of cooked meat per portion.
3. Beef and noodles may be prepared in the morning and refrigerated until later if desired. Bake 1 hour in step 5 if mixture is put directly from the refrigerator into the oven.

DIETARY INFORMATION
May be used as written by general, no added salt, low fat, low cholesterol and mechanical soft diets. Diabetic diets — each serving provides 2 bread and 3 medium fat meat exchanges. Bland diets — omit pepper. Each serving provides 2 ounces cooked beef.

Beef with Noodles and Olives

Refer to footnotes for special dietary information

INGREDIENTS	WEIGHTS/MEASURES	YIELD ADJUST.	METHOD
Noodles . . . . .4 pounds Boiling water . . . . .4 gallons Salt . . . . .¼ cup Vegetable oil . . . . .2 tablespoons			1. Drop noodles into boiling, salted water; stir lightly to mix; add oil; cook, uncovered, about 15 minutes or until tender; rinse well with cold water.
Chopped onions . . . . .1 quart Margarine . . . . .¼ cup (2 ounces) Ground beef . . . . .8 pounds, 12 ounces			2. Fry onions in margarine in pot until golden; add ground beef; cook and stir over medium heat until meat is broken up and browned; pour meat into a colander; drain off fat and liquid; discard fat and liquid; return meat to the pot.
Tomato puree . . . . .3 quarts (1 No. 10 can) Tomato juice . . . . .1 quart Garlic powder . . . . .2 teaspoons Dried parsley flakes . . . . .¼ cup Basil .2 teaspoons Salt . . . . .¼ cup Pepper . . . . .1 teaspoon			3. Add tomato puree, tomato juice, garlic, parsley, basil, salt and pepper to meat; bring to a boil; reduce heat; cover and simmer over low heat for 45 minutes, stirring occasionally.
Chopped pimiento-stuffed salad-type green olives . . . . .1½ quarts			4. Add olives and noodles to meat mixture; mix lightly. Pour half of the mixture into each of 2 greased steam table pans. 5. Cover pans with aluminum foil; bake 30 minutes. Serve hot.

Beef Patties with Cheese

Refer to footnotes for special dietary information

INGREDIENTS	WEIGHTS/MEASURES	YIELD ADJUST.	METHOD
Dill seed . . . . .2 tablespoons Water. .2 cups Salad mustard. . . . . .½ cup Salt . . . . .2 tablespoons Pepper. . . . . .1 teaspoon Sliced day-old bread . . . . .1 pound			1. Soak dill seed in water in mixer bowl for 30 minutes; add mustard, salt, pepper and bread; mix 1 minute at low speed.
Ground beef . . . . .13 pounds Coarsely grated or chopped cheddar cheese . . . . .1 pound			2. Add beef and cheese to bread mixture; mix 2 to 3 minutes at medium speed. 3. Use a rounded No. 12 dipper to shape meat into 5-ounce meat rounds; flatten round to about 4 inches in diameter. 4. Bake 15 to 20 minutes or until center is no longer pink.

YIELD
50 portions

PORTION SIZE
1 patty

PAN SIZE
18 × 26-inch sheet pans

TEMPERATURE
375°F. Oven

DIETARY INFORMATION
May be used as written for general, no added salt, low fat and mechanical soft diets. Diabetic diets — each serving provides 3½ lean meat and 1 vegetable exchanges. Bland diets — omit pepper. Each serving provides 3½ ounces beef and cheese.

YIELD
50 portions (4 loaves)

PORTION SIZE
4 ounces

PAN SIZE
18 × 26-inch sheet pan

TEMPERATURE
325°F. Oven

DIETARY INFORMATION
May be used as written for general, bland, no added salt and mechanical soft diets. Diabetic diets — each serving provides 3 medium fat meat, 1/2 bread and 1 fat exchanges. Each serving provides 3 ounces cooked beef.

Madrid Meat Loaf

Refer to footnotes for special dietary information

INGREDIENTS	WEIGHTS/MEASURES	YIELD ADJUST.	METHOD
Lean ground beef . . . . .12 pounds, 4 ounces			1. Put all ingredients in a mixer bowl in the order shown; mix at low speed, using beater, about 3 minutes or until well blended. DO NOT OVERMIX.
Nonfat dry milk . . . . .2⅔ cups			2. Remove mixture from mixer; shape into 4 equal loaves; put loaves on a lightly greased sheet pan; bake 1½ to 1¾ hours or until browned and firm.
Eggs .2 cups (10-12 medium)			3. Let loaves set 10 to 15 minutes and then slice into 4-ounce portions. (12 to 13 slices per loaf.)
Finely chopped onions . . . . . . .2 cups			
Chopped pimiento-stuffed salad-style green olives . . . .1 quart			
Salt . . . . .3 tablespoons			
Dry parsley flakes . . . . .3 tablespoons			
Rolled oats . . . . .1 quart			
Water. . . . . .1 quart			

Meat Balls

Refer to footnotes for special dietary information

INGREDIENTS	WEIGHTS/MEASURES	YIELD ADJUST.	METHOD
Sliced day-old white bread . . . . 1 pound Water. . . . . .3 cups			1. Put bread and water in a mixer bowl; mix 1 minute at low speed.
Finely chopped onions . . . . . . .1 cup Finely chopped celery . . . . . . .1½ cups Lean ground beef . . . . .6 pounds Lean ground pork . . . . .3 pounds Salt . . . . .1½ tablespoons Worcestershire sauce. . . . . . . .2 tablespoons Eggs . . . . .1½ cups (8 to 9 medium)			2. Add onions, celery, beef, pork, salt, Worcestershire sauce and eggs to the bread; mix 3 minutes at low speed or until blended. 3. Shape meat mixture gently into 2-ounce balls using a No. 20 dipper to portion the meat. Weigh several meat balls to check weight. 4. Put meat balls on lightly greased sheet pan; bake 45 minutes or until browned and firm.

YIELD
50 portions (100 meat balls)

PORTION SIZE
2 meat balls

PAN SIZE
18 × 26-inch sheet pan

TEMPERATURE
350°F. Oven

NOTES
1. 8 pounds, 8 ounces ground lean beef may be used instead of beef and pork in step 2.
2. Lean ground beef should be used in this recipe. If regular ground beef is used, meat balls should be browned in a roasting pan because the sheet pan will not hold all of the fat which will cook out of the meat balls.

DIETARY INFORMATION
May be used as written for general, no added salt, bland, and mechanical soft diets. Diabetic diets — each serving of 2 meat balls provides 2 lean meat and 1 vegetable exchanges. Each serving provides 2 ounces of cooked beef.

YIELD
50 portions (4 loaves)

PORTION SIZE
4½ ounces

PAN SIZE
18 × 26-inch sheet pans

TEMPERATURE
350°F. Oven

DIETARY INFORMATION
May be used as written for general, no added salt and mechanical soft diets. Diabetic diets — each serving provides 1 bread and 3 lean meat exchanges. Bland diets — omit pepper. Each serving provides 3 ounces of cooked beef.

Meat Loaf

Refer to footnotes for special dietary information

INGREDIENTS	WEIGHTS/MEASURES	YIELD ADJUST.	METHOD
Eggs	1 quart (20-24 medium)		1. Whip eggs at moderate speed in mixer bowl for ½ minute.
Nonfat dry milk	1½ cups		2. Stir milk into very hot water; water should be almost but not quite boiling; pour hot milk into the eggs, beating constantly at moderate speed; stop mixer; remove whip and substitute beater for the remaining mixing.
Very hot water	1 quart		
Ground lean beef	9 pounds		3. Add beef, pork, tomato juice, salt, pepper, chopped onions and bread crumbs to eggs; mix 2 to 3 minutes at slow speed or until well mixed.
Ground lean pork	2 pounds		4. Remove mixture from mixer; shape into 4 equal loaves; put loaves on a lightly greased sheet pan; bake 1½ to 1¾ hours or until browned and firm.
Tomato juice	2 cups		5. Let loaves set 10 to 15 minutes and then slice into 4½ ounce portions. (12 to 13 slices per loaf.)
Salt	¼ cup		
Pepper	½ teaspoon		
Chopped onions	2 cups		
Dry bread crumbs	2 pounds (2 quarts)		

Meat Sauce for Spaghetti

Refer to footnotes for special dietary information

INGREDIENTS	WEIGHTS/MEASURES	YIELD ADJUST.	METHOD
Finely chopped celery . . . . . . .1½ quarts Finely chopped onions. . . . . . .1½ quarts Vegetable oil . . . . .¼ cup			1. Brown celery and onions in oil in heavy pot, stirring occasionally, until onions are golden.
Ground beef . . . . .4 pounds, 6 ounces			2. Add ground beef to vegetables; cook and stir over moderate heat until meat is broken up and well browned. 3. Drain meat and vegetables well in a colander; discard fat; return meat and vegetables to pot.
Tomato puree . . . . .4½ quarts (1½ No. 10 cans) Salt. .¼ cup Sugar. . . . . .¼ cup Tomato juice . . . . .1 quart			4. Add tomato puree, salt, sugar and tomato juice; mix well and cook, uncovered, over low heat, stirring occasionally, for 1½ hours. (The sauce should just be barely simmering.)
Ground oregano . . . . .1 teaspoon Garlic powder . . . . .1 teaspoon Ground cloves. . . . . .½ teaspoon Ground thyme. . . . . .1 teaspoon Basil . . . . .½ teaspoon Hot beef stock . . . . .as necessary			5. Add oregano, garlic, cloves, thyme and basil to sauce; mix well and simmer, stirring occasionally, for another 30 minutes. Add beef stock, a cup at a time, if sauce gets too thick. 6. Serve over hot, well-drained spaghetti.

YIELD
50 portions (about 1½ gallons)

PORTION SIZE
½ cup (4-ounce ladle)

PAN SIZE
Heavy 3-gallon pot

NOTES
1. This sauce is best if made the day before it is served and refrigerated overnight to give the seasoning a chance to develop flavor.
2. This is a mild sauce. If a spicier sauce is desired, it is suggested that the amounts of oregano and garlic powder be increased to 2 teaspoons each.
3. The amount of beef may be increased to 8 pounds, 12 ounces if it is to be served without meat balls. 8 pounds, 12 ounces of beef would provide 2 ounces of meat per person.

DIETARY INFORMATION
May be used as written for general, no added salt, low cholesterol and mechanical soft diets. Diabetic diets — each serving provides 1 lean meat and 1 bread exchanges, for the sauce without any spaghetti. Bland diets — omit cloves. Each serving provides 1 ounce of cooked beef.

YIELD
50 portions (100 meat balls)

PORTION SIZE
2 meat balls

PAN SIZE
18 × 26-inch sheet pans
Roasting pan

TEMPERATURE
350°F. Oven

NOTE
Lean ground beef should be used in this recipe. If regular ground beef is used, meat balls should be browned in a roasting pan because the sheet pan will not hold all of the fat which will cook out of the meat balls.

DIETARY INFORMATION
May be used as written for general, no added salt, bland and mechanical soft diets. Diabetic diets — each serving provides 3 lean meat and 1 bread exchanges. Each serving provides 3 ounces cooked beef and eggs.

Porcupine Meat Balls

Refer to footnotes for special dietary information

INGREDIENTS	WEIGHTS/MEASURES	YIELD ADJUST.	METHOD
Lean ground beef . . . . .13 pounds Long grain rice . . . . .1½ pounds (about 3½ cups) Slightly beaten eggs . . . . .2 cups (10 to 12 medium) Finely chopped onions . . . . . . .1 quart Salt .2 tablespoons Water. . . . . .1 quart			1. Put ground beef in mixer bowl; add rice, eggs, onions, salt and water; mix at low speed 2 to 4 minutes or until well blended. DO NOT OVERMIX. 2. Shape gently into 3-ounce meat balls using a No. 12 dipper to portion meat. Weigh several meat balls to check weight. 3. Put meat balls on lightly greased sheet pans and bake 45 minutes; drain off fat and transfer meat balls to roasting pan.
Tomato puree . . . . .3 quarts (1 No. 10 can) Water. . . . . .3 quarts Oregano . . . . .1 tablespoon Basil .1 teaspoon Garlic granules . . . . .1 teaspoon Salt .2 tablespoons			4. Combine tomato puree, water, oregano, basil, garlic and salt; bring to a simmer and pour over hot meat balls. 5. Bake 45 minutes, covered, or until rice is tender.

Salisbury Steak

Refer to footnotes for special dietary information

INGREDIENTS	WEIGHTS/MEASURES	YIELD ADJUST.	METHOD
Sliced day-old bread . . . . .1 pound 8 ounces Milk . . . . .1 quart			1. Combine bread and milk in mixer bowl; beat 1 minute at low speed.
Finely chopped onions . . . . . . .3 cups Salt . . . . .2 tablespoons Tomato catsup . . . . .2 cups Lean ground beef . . . . .13 pounds			2. Add onions, salt, catsup and beef to bread mixture; mix 2 to 3 minutes at low speed or until well mixed. DO NOT OVERMIX. 3. Shape meat mixture into 5 to 6-ounce oval patties; put on lightly greased baking sheet and bake 1 hour or until firm and center is no longer pink.

YIELD
50 portions

PORTION SIZE
1 steak

PAN SIZE
18 × 26-inch sheet pan

TEMPERATURE
350°F. Oven

DIETARY INFORMATION
May be used as written for general, bland, no added salt and mechanical soft diets. Diabetic diets — each serving provides 1/2 bread and 3 lean meat exchanges. Each serving provides 3 ounces of cooked beef.

YIELD
50 portions (2 pans)

PORTION SIZE
¾ cup (6 ounces)
plus potatoes

PAN SIZE
Heavy 5-gallon pot
12 × 20 × 2-inch steam table pans

TEMPERATURE
350°F. Oven

NOTE
The pies may be prepared earlier in the day and refrigerated until needed. Baking time should be increased to 45 minutes or until potatoes are browned and the pie is hot.

DIETARY INFORMATION
May be used as written for general, no added salt, low cholesterol and mechanical soft diets. Diabetic diets — each serving provides 2 lean meat, 1 bread and 1 vegetable exchanges. Bland diets — omit pepper. Each serving provides 2 ounces cooked beef.

Shepherd's Pie

Refer to footnotes for special dietary information

INGREDIENTS	WEIGHTS/MEASURES	YIELD ADJUST.	METHOD
Chopped onions	3 cups		1. Fry onions in margarine in pot until golden; add ground beef; cook and stir over medium heat until meat is broken up and well browned; pour meat into a colander; drain off as much fat as possible; discard fat and return meat to pot.
Margarine	¼ cup (½ stick)		
Ground beef	8 pounds, 12 ounces		
Salt	3 tablespoons		2. Add salt, pepper, carrots and tomatoes to meat and simmer, covered, about 20 minutes or until carrots are tender.
Pepper	1 teaspoon		
Diced raw carrots	1 quart		
Canned, crushed tomatoes	3 quarts (1 No. 10 can)		
All-purpose flour	1½ cups		3. Stir flour and water together to form a smooth paste; stir paste into hot meat mixture; cook and stir over moderate heat until thickened.
Water	1½ cups		
Canned drained peas	3 quarts (1 No. 10 can)		4. Add canned peas to meat mixture; simmer, uncovered, another 10 minutes, stirring occasionally. Pour ½ of the mixture into each of 2 steam table pans.
Mashed potatoes	1 gallon		5. Put 25 scant No. 12 scoops of potatoes on top of meat in each pan; bake 15 minutes or until potatoes are lightly browned.

Sloppy Joe on a Bun

Refer to footnotes for special dietary information

INGREDIENTS	WEIGHTS/MEASURES	YIELD ADJUST.	METHOD
Finely chopped onions........1 quart Finely chopped celery ....1 quart Vegetable oil..............¼ cup			1. Fry onions and celery in oil in pot until onions are golden.
Ground beef..............8 pounds, 12 ounces			2. Add ground beef to vegetables; cook and stir over moderate heat until meat is broken up and well browned. 3. Drain meat and vegetables well in a colander; discard fat; return meat and vegetables to pot.
Tomato sauce..............1¼ gallons (1⅔ No. 10 cans) Tomato catsup.............2 cups Salt....................2 tablespoons Pepper...................1 teaspoon Ground thyme.............½ teaspoon Basil....................1 tablespoon			4. Add tomato sauce, catsup, salt, pepper, thyme and basil to the meat. Simmer, uncovered, stirring frequently, 20 to 25 minutes.
Hamburger buns...........50			5. Serve ½ cup of the meat mixture on bottom half of each bun; cover with top half of bun and serve hot.

YIELD
50 portions (about 1½ gallons)

PORTION SIZE
½ cup (4-ounce ladle)
plus bun

PAN SIZE
Heavy 3-gallon pot

DIETARY INFORMATION
May be used as written for general, no added salt, low cholesterol and mechanical soft diets. Diabetic diets — each serving provides 2 lean meat and 2 vegetable exchanges. Bland diets — omit pepper. Each serving provides 2 ounces of cooked beef.

YIELD
50 portions (100 meat balls)

PORTION SIZE
2 meat balls plus gravy

PAN SIZE
18 × 26-inch sheet pan
Roasting pan

TEMPERATURE
350°F. Oven

NOTE
Lean ground beef should be used in this recipe. If regular ground beef is used, meat balls should be browned in a roasting pan because the sheet pan will not hold all of the fat which will cook out of the meat balls.

DIETARY INFORMATION
May be used as written for general, no added salt and mechanical soft diets.
Diabetic diets — each serving provides 3 lean meat and 1 bread exchanges.
Bland diets — omit pepper and nutmeg.
Each serving provides 3 ounces of cooked beef.

Swedish Meat Balls

Refer to footnotes for special dietary information

INGREDIENTS	WEIGHTS/MEASURES	YIELD ADJUST.	METHOD
Dry bread crumbs . . . . .1 pound, 8 ounces (1½ quarts) Water. . . . . .3 cups			1. Put bread crumbs and water in mixer bowl; mix 1 minute at low speed.
Lean ground beef . . . . .12 pounds Slightly beaten eggs. . . . . . . .2 cups (10-12 medium) Salt .¼ cup Pepper. . . . . .1 teaspoon Ground nutmeg. . . . . .1½ tablespoons			2. Add beef, eggs, salt, pepper and nutmeg to crumbs; mix at low speed 2 to 3 minutes or until blended. 3. Shape gently into 2½-ounce balls using a No. 16 dipper to portion the meat. Weigh several meat balls to check weight. 4. Put meat balls on lightly greased sheet pan; bake 45 minutes or until browned and firm; transfer meat balls to roasting pan.
Milk .3 quarts All-purpose flour . . . . .1½ cups Salt .2 teaspoons Pepper. . . . . .¼ teaspoon			5. Pour as much fat as possible off sheet pan; use 2 quarts of milk to wash the drippings off the sheet pan into a saucepan; scrape any brown particles remaining on the pan into the saucepan with the milk. 6. Make a smooth paste of the remaining 1 quart of milk, flour, salt and pepper; add paste to drippings and milk and cook and stir over low heat until smooth and thickened; add cold water if gravy is too thick; stir until smooth; pour gravy over meat balls; cover; bake about 45 minutes.

Stuffed Green Peppers

Refer to footnotes for special dietary information

INGREDIENTS	WEIGHTS/MEASURES	YIELD ADJUST.	METHOD
Fresh green peppers.........25 large or 50 medium Boiling water...............as necessary			1. Wash peppers, cut each pepper in half lengthwise; remove core. If peppers are small, core and use whole pepper. 2. Cover peppers with boiling water; bring to a boil; cook 1 minute. DO NOT OVERCOOK. Drain peppers right away and set aside for use in step 4.
Lean ground beef ....13 pounds Finely chopped onions.......1 quart Rolled oats ....5 cups Pepper....................1 teaspoon Salt ....1/4 cup Worcestershire sauce........3/4 cup Tomato juice ....3 cups Water....................3 cups			3. Combine beef, onions, oatmeal, pepper, salt, Worcestershire sauce, tomato juice and water; mix only until blended; do not overmix. 4. Fill each pepper with 2/3 cup (2 level No. 12 dippers) mixture. Put peppers in roasting pans.
Hot water ....as necessary			5. Pour about 1/2 inch hot water in bottom of each roasting pan; cover tightly and bake about 2 hours or until peppers are tender and filling is firm and browned.

YIELD
50 portions

PORTION SIZE
1 stuffed pepper

PAN SIZE
Roasting pans

TEMPERATURE
350°F. Oven

DIETARY INFORMATION
May be used as written for general, no added salt and mechanical soft diets. Diabetic diets — each serving provides 3 1/2 medium fat meat and 1/2 bread exchanges. Each serving provides 3 ounces cooked beef.

YIELD
50 portions (2 pans)

PORTION SIZE
¾ cup (6 ounces)

PAN SIZE
Heavy 8-quart pot
12 × 20 × 2-inch steam table pans

TEMPERATURE
350°F. Oven

VARIATION
Baked chicken and dressing. Substitute chicken and chicken broth for beef and broth in steps 1 and 3.

NOTE
Beef trimmings and drippings from roast beef may be substituted for canned beef and broth in steps 1 and 3. Dressing should be baked to the consistency for dressing most popular in your area.

DIETARY INFORMATION
May be used as written for general, and no added salt diets. Diabetic diets — each serving provides 2 bread, 2½ medium fat meat and 1 fat exchanges. Bland diets — omit pepper. Each serving provides 2 ounces of cooked beef.

Baked Beef and Dressing

Refer to footnotes for special dietary information

INGREDIENTS	WEIGHTS/MEASURES	YIELD ADJUST.	METHOD
Canned beef	.6 pounds, 4 ounces (1 No. 10 can)		1. Place beef and juice in colander. Drain juice from meat. Skim off any fat from juice and remove any visible fat from meat. Cover and set aside for later use. Refrigerate if not to be used within 30 minutes.
Margarine	.2 cups (1 pound)		2. Place ½ cup margarine in pot. Add celery and onions and cook and stir over moderate heat until onions are soft but not browned. Add remaining margarine so that margarine will melt in the pot.
Chopped celery	.1½ quarts		
Chopped onions	.1½ quarts		
Fat-free beef stock	.as necessary		3. Add as much beef broth as necessary to beef juice to yield 1 gallon liquid. Add to vegetables in pot. Cool to room temperature, if necessary. Add eggs, pepper and sage to mixture. Taste for seasoning and add more salt, if necessary. (The amount of salt necessary will depend upon the saltiness of the broth.)
Slightly beaten eggs	.2 cups (10 to 12 medium)		
Pepper	.1 teaspoon		
Sage	.2 tablespoons		
Salt	.as necessary		
Diced, day-old white or whole wheat bread	.3 gallons (6 pounds)		4. Place bread in mixer bowl. Add reserved meat and vegetable broth mixture. Mix at low speed only until blended. 5. Place ½ of the mixture in each of 2 well-greased pans. Bake 1¼ to 1½ hours or until lightly browned. Serve hot, with gravy, if desired.

Roast Veal

Refer to footnotes for special dietary information

INGREDIENTS	WEIGHTS/MEASURES	YIELD ADJUST.	METHOD

Boneless veal roast
  (rolled leg or shoulder) . . . . .14 pounds,
                  8 ounces
Salt . . . . .3 tablespoons
Pepper. . . . . .1½ teaspoons
			1. Rub each roast with salt and pepper.
			2. Place roasts in roasting pan without crowding; do not cover pan or add water.
			3. Insert a meat thermometer in thickest part of meat; cook meat until meat thermometer registers 170°F or cook 2¼ to 3½ hours depending upon size of roast.
			4. Remove meat from roaster; cool 20 to 30 minutes before it is sliced. (If meat is not to be used right away, it should be refrigerated after it has cooled for 30 minutes.)
			5. Use any drippings for making gravy. If gravy is not to be made for that meal, drippings should be refrigerated until used. (Scrape brown particles from pan and use with drippings for gravy.)

YIELD
50 portions

PORTION SIZE
3 ounces

PAN SIZE
Roasting pan

TEMPERATURE
325°F. Oven

NOTE
If frozen roast are used, they should be cooked 3¼ to 4½ hours.

DIETARY INFORMATION
May be used as written for general, soft, no added salt, low fat and low cholesterol diets. Diabetic diets — each serving provides 3 lean meat exchanges. Bland and restricted residue diets — omit pepper. Each serving provides 3 ounces cooked veal.

YIELD
50 portions (3 pans)

PORTION SIZE
1 cutlet plus
2 tablespoons sauce

PAN SIZE
18 × 26-inch sheet pans
12 × 20 × 2-inch steam table pans

TEMPERATURE
325°F. Oven

VARIATION
Baked Veal Cutlets with Mushroom Sauce: Use cream of mushroom soup instead of cream of tomato soup in step 4.

DIETARY INFORMATION
May be used as written for general, no added salt, and low cholesterol diets. Diabetic diets — each serving provides 1 bread and 3 lean meat exchanges. Bland diets — omit pepper. Each serving provides 3 ounces cooked veal.

Veal Cutlets with Tomato Sauce

Refer to footnotes for special dietary information

INGREDIENTS	WEIGHTS/MEASURES	YIELD ADJUST.	METHOD
All-purpose flour	2 quarts		1. Sift flour, onion salt, salt, garlic powder, pepper and thyme together into a shallow pan.
Onion salt	1 tablespoon		
Salt	2 tablespoons		
Garlic powder	2 teaspoons		
Pepper	1 teaspoon		
Ground thyme	1 teaspoon		
Vegetable oil	as necessary		2. Put oil in a shallow pan; dip cutlets in oil; drain well in a colander.
Veal cutlets	12 pounds, 8 ounces (50 4-ounce cutlets)		3. Dredge well-drained cutlets in flour mixture; put on well-greased pans in a single layer; bake 30 minutes or until browned. Arrange browned cutlets shingle style in steam table pans.
Nonfat dry milk	1 cup		4. Stir dry milk into water; add to soup; stir until smooth; pour ⅓ of the soup mixture over cutlets in each steam table pan.
Warm water	3 cups		
Canned cream of tomato soup	1 46-ounce can		5. Cover pans with aluminum foil; bake about 45 minutes or until cutlets are tender.

Veal Paprika

Refer to footnotes for special dietary information

INGREDIENTS	WEIGHTS/MEASURES	YIELD ADJUST.	METHOD
Margarine . . . . .½ cup (4 ounces) Boneless veal stew meat . . . . .14 pounds Paprika . . . . .½ cup All-purpose flour . . . . .1 cup Salt .¼ cup			1. Grease roaster heavily using all of the margarine; put veal in roaster. 2. Combine paprika, flour and salt and sprinkle over meat; stir lightly to mix well.
Chopped onions . . . . .1 quart			3. Sprinkle onions over meat; roast, uncovered, about 1 hour or until meat is browned.
Hot water . . . . .3 quarts			4. Pour water over meat; cover and bake about 1 hour longer or until meat is tender. Put roasting pan on top of the range after veal is tender.
Sour cream (room temperature) . . . . .2 quarts			5. Stir sour cream into meat and gravy; reheat over low heat but do not let boil after cream is added. Serve hot.

YIELD
50 portions (about 2 gallons)

PORTION SIZE
5 ounces

PAN SIZE
Roasting pan

TEMPERATURE
350°F. Oven

DIETARY INFORMATION
May be used as written for general, bland, and no added salt diets. Diabetic diets — each serving provides 3½ medium fat meat, 1 vegetable and 1 fat exchanges. Each serving provides 3 ounces cooked veal.

YIELD
50 portions (2 pans)

PORTION SIZE
1 cup (8 ounces)

PAN SIZE
Roasting pan
12 × 20 × 2-inch steam table pans

TEMPERATURE
350°F. Oven

DIETARY INFORMATION
May be used as written for general, no added salt, and low cholesterol diets. Diabetic diets — each serving provides 4 high fat meat and 1 bread exchanges. Bland diets — omit pepper. Each serving provides 3 ounces cooked veal.

Veal and Noodle Casserole

Refer to footnotes for special dietary information

INGREDIENTS	WEIGHTS/MEASURES	YIELD ADJUST.	METHOD
Canned mushrooms . . . . .3 16-ounce cans			1. Drain and chop mushrooms; keep juice for use in step 3.
Veal shoulder, cut into 1-inch cubes . . . . . .14 pounds, 4 ounces Minced garlic . . . . .3 cloves Chopped onions . . . . .1 quart Salt .2 tablespoons Pepper. . . . . .½ teaspoon Margarine . . . . .½ cup (4 ounces)			2. Put veal in roasting pan; sprinkle with garlic, onions, salt and pepper; dot with butter or margarine; cover and bake, stirring occasionally, 1 hour or until veal is tender. Put roasting pan on top of range after veal is tender.
Egg noodles . . . . .2 pounds, 8 ounces (3¾ quarts) Boiling water. . . . . .2 gallons Salt .2 tablespoons Vegetable oil . . . . .2 tablespoons			3. Add noodles to boiling salted water. Add oil and cook, stirring occasionally, about 12 minutes or until noodles are tender; drain noodles but do not rinse them. Try to have noodles cooked and hot about the time veal is ready.
Liquid from mushrooms . . . . . .as available Dry white table wine (optional) . . . . .2 cups Water. . . . . .2 quarts Worcestershire sauce . . . . . . .2 tablespoons All-purpose flour . . . . .1 cup Paprika . . . . .1 tablespoon Salt .2 tablespoons Pepper. . . . . .½ teaspoon Cold water. . . . . .2 cups			4. Add the mushroom liquid, wine, water and Worcestershire sauce to the meat. Stir flour, paprika, salt and pepper into cold water to form a smooth paste. Pour flour mixture into meat mixture and cook and stir over medium heat until smooth and thickened.
Sour cream or yogurt (room temperature) . . . . .1 quart Grated Parmesan cheese . . . . .1 cup			5. Add mushrooms and noodles to veal; stir sour cream or yogurt into mixture; pour ½ of the mixture into each of 2 buttered steam table pans. 6. Sprinkle ½ of the cheese over each pan; bake for 45 mins.

Baked Canned Ham

Refer to footnotes for special dietary information

INGREDIENTS	WEIGHTS/MEASURES	YIELD ADJUST.	METHOD
Canned ham . . . . .15 pounds			1. Trim ham and slice into 100 slices 2 ounces each. Put the slices back together in the shape of the ham. Put each ham on a piece of aluminum foil large enough to bring it up around the ham to form a tight collar of aluminum foil. Leave the top of the ham open and shape the collar so that it comes about ½ inch above the top of the ham. (It is not necessary to tie the ham but if it has been sliced and tied, it may be left tied until it is served.) Put hams into roasting pan.
Brown sugar . . . . .3 cups Vinegar . . . . .1 cup Ground cloves. . . . . .1 tablespoon			2. Combine sugar, vinegar and cloves; mix until smooth; put an equal amount of the sugar mixture on top of each ham. 3. Insert a meat thermometer in the center of the largest ham and bake, uncovered, until the thermometer registers 140°F. or Bake, uncovered, about 1½ to 2 hours. (The length of time will depend upon the size of the hams.

YIELD
50 portions

PORTION SIZE
2 slices (3 ounces)

PAN SIZE
Roaster

TEMPERATURE
325°F. Oven

NOTE
Other glazes may be used for the ham instead of the brown sugar, vinegar and cloves.

DIETARY INFORMATION
May be used as written for general and no added salt diets. Diabetic diets — bake ham without sugar, vinegar and cloves. Each serving yields 3 medium fat meat exchanges. Bland diets — omit cloves. Each serving provides 3 ounces cooked ham.

YIELD
50 portions

PORTION SIZE
3 ounces (2 slices)

PAN SIZE
18 × 26-inch sheet pan

TEMPERATURE
325°F. Oven

DIETARY INFORMATION
May be used as written for general, bland, and no added salt diets. Diabetic diets — each serving provides 3 medium fat exchanges without the sugar, vinegar, water and mustard sauce. Each serving provides 3 ounces cooked ham.

Glazed Ham Slices

Refer to footnotes for special dietary information

INGREDIENTS WEIGHTS/MEASURES	YIELD ADJUST.	METHOD
Canned ham . . . . .15 pounds		1. Trim and slice ham into 100 slices about 2 ounces each. Put slices on a sheet pan partially covering each other in shingled style.
Brown sugar . . . . .2¾ cups Vinegar . . . . .½ cup Water. .¼ cup Salad mustard. . . . . .2 tablespoons		2. Combine sugar, vinegar, water and mustard; mix well; pour evenly over ham slices. 3. Bake about 30 minutes or until ham is hot and glazed.

Ham a la King

Refer to footnotes for special dietary information

INGREDIENTS	WEIGHTS/MEASURES	YIELD ADJUST.	METHOD
Canned mushrooms	2 1-pound cans		1. Drain mushrooms; keep juice for use in step 2; chop mushrooms coarsely.
Nonfat dry milk . . . . Juice from the mushrooms and hot water	5½ cups 1 gallon		2. Stir milk into water; mix well; cool to lukewarm.
Margarine . . . . All-purpose flour	1 cup (8 ounces) 1½ cups		3. Fry mushrooms in margarine over moderate heat about 5 minutes; stir flour into mixture; cook and stir over low heat until smooth. 4. Add milk to mushroom mixture; cook and stir over moderate heat until smooth and thickened; continue to cook over low heat, stirring occasionally, until the starchy taste is gone.
Chopped hard-cooked eggs . . . Diced cooked ham . . . . Chopped pimientos . . . . Sherry (optional) . . . . Salt	12 5 pounds, 8 ounces 1 cup 1 cup as necessary		5. Add eggs, ham, pimientos and sherry to hot sauce; add salt, if necessary. 6. Reheat over low heat and serve hot.

YIELD
50 portions (about 2¼ gallons)

PORTION SIZE
¾ cup (6-ounce ladle)

PAN SIZE
Heavy 3-gallon pot

DIETARY INFORMATION
May be used as written for general, no added salt, and bland diets. Diabetic diets — each serving provides 2 lean meat and ½ bread exchanges. Each serving provides 2 ounces cooked ham and eggs.

YIELD
50 portions (2 pans)

PORTION SIZE
¾ cup (6 ounces)

PAN SIZE
Heavy 3-gallon pot
12 × 20 × 2-inch steam table pans

TEMPERATURE
375°F. Oven

NOTES
1. 14 pounds, 8 ounces fresh white potatoes will yield approximately 12 pounds, 8 ounces peeled potatoes.
2. 2 pounds dehydrated sliced potatoes can be cooked 15 to 25 minutes or until tender and used instead of the potatoes in step 1.

DIETARY INFORMATION
May be used as written for general and no added salt diets. Diabetic diets — each serving provides 2 high fat meat and 1½ bread exchanges. Bland diets — omit pepper. Each serving provides 2 ounces cooked ham.

Scalloped Potatoes and Ham

Refer to footnotes for special dietary information

INGREDIENTS	WEIGHTS/MEASURES	YIELD ADJUST.	METHOD
Fresh white thinly sliced potatoes	12 pounds, 8 ounces		1. Cover potatoes with boiling water; add salt; bring to a boil; cook 10 minutes or just until barely tender; drain well.
Boiling water	as necessary		2. Put half of the drained potatoes into each of 2 well-greased pans.
Salt	1 tablespoon		
Nonfat dry milk	2 quarts		3. Stir milk into water; mix well; heat milk to just below the boiling point but do not let it boil.
Warm water	1½ gallons		
Margarine, melted	1½ cups (12 ounces)		4. Mix melted margarine with flour and pepper; stir until smooth; add to hot milk; cook and stir over low heat until smooth and thickened.
All-purpose flour	1½ cups		
Pepper	1 teaspoon		
Diced canned ham	6 pounds, 4 ounces		5. Add ham to hot sauce; stir lightly; pour half of the ham and sauce over potatoes in each pan; stir lightly to mix potatoes, ham and sauce together. 6. Bake 1 hour or until lightly browned.

Ham and Egg Souffle

Refer to footnotes for special dietary information

INGREDIENTS	WEIGHTS/MEASURES	YIELD ADJUST.	METHOD
Eggs . . . . .3 cups (15 to 18 medium)			1. Place eggs in mixer bowl and mix at low speed about ½ minute to blend lightly.
Skim milk . . . . .1½ quarts Cubed fresh white bread. . . . . .6 slices (6 ounces) Grated cheddar cheese . . . . . .1 quart (1 pound) Chopped ham trimmings with all visible fat removed. . . . . .1½ quarts (2 pounds) Salt .2 teaspoons			2. Add milk, bread, cheese, ham and salt to the eggs and mix lightly. (The bread should still be in cubes.) Pour into well-greased pan; cover and refrigerate overnight. 3. Bake 1 hour. Remove from heat and cut 4 × 8. Serve hot for breakfast, brunch, or lunch.

YIELD
32 portions (1 pan)

PORTION SIZE
1 square

PAN SIZE
12 × 18-inch cake pan

TEMPERATURE
350°F. Oven

NOTE
3 pounds of pork sausage, cooked, drained and crumbled or 3 pounds of bacon, cooked, drained and crumbled may be substituted for the ham trimmings.

DIETARY INFORMATION
May be used as written for general and bland diets. Diabetic diets — each serving provides 1 medium fat meat and ⅓ bread exchanges. Each serving provides 1 ounce meat and cheese.

YIELD
50 portions

PORTION SIZE
3 ounces

PAN SIZE
Roasting pan

TEMPERATURE
325°F. Oven

NOTE
If frozen roasts are used they should be cooked as follows:
Rolled loin: 3 to 4¼ hours.
Rolled shoulder: 4 to 5 hours.
Rolled fresh ham: 5¾ to 6½ hours.

DIETARY INFORMATION
May be used as written for general and no added salt diets. Diabetic diets — each serving provides 3 medium fat meat exchanges. Bland and restricted residue diets — omit pepper. Low fat and low cholesterol diets — remove all visible fat before cooking. Each serving provides 3 ounces cooked pork.

Roast Pork

Refer to footnotes for special dietary information

INGREDIENTS	WEIGHTS/MEASURES	YIELD ADJUST.	METHOD
Boneless pork roast (rolled loin, shoulder or fresh ham) . . . . 15 pounds Salt . . . . ¼ cup Pepper . . . . 1 tablespoon			1. Rub outside of meat with salt and pepper. 2. Place roasts in pan without crowding; do not cover pan or add water. 3. Insert meat thermometer in center of the thickest part of one of the rolls and cook until meat thermometer registers 180°F. <div align="center">or</div>Cook rolled loin (3 to 5 pounds) 2 to 3¼ hours. Cook rolled shoulder (5 to 8 pounds) 3 to 4 hours. Cook rolled fresh ham (10 to 14 pounds) 4¾ to 5½ hours. 4. Remove meat from the pan; cool 20 to 30 minutes before slicing. (If meat is not to be used immediately, it should be refrigerated after 30 minutes.)

Braised Pork Chops

Refer to footnotes for special dietary information

INGREDIENTS	WEIGHTS/MEASURES	YIELD ADJUST.	METHOD
Pork chops	17 pounds, 8 ounces (50 chops about 5 ounces each)		1. Put chops on lightly greased sheet pans; bake 1 hour; pour off as much fat as possible. 2. Put 25 chops, shingle style, in each of 2 steam table pans.
Hot water . . . . Salt . . . . Thyme	1 quart 2 tablespoons 2 teaspoons		3. Pour 2 cups hot water over chops in each pan; sprinkle salt and thyme on chops; cover with aluminum foil; bake 1 hour or until tender.

YIELD
50 portions (2 pans)

PORTION SIZE
1 chop

PAN SIZE
18 × 26-inch sheet pans
12 × 20 × 2-inch steam table pans

TEMPERATURE
350°F. Oven

DIETARY INFORMATION
May be used as written for general, no added salt, bland, low fat and restricted residue diets. Diabetic diets — each serving provides 3 medium fat meat exchanges. Each serving provides 3 ounces cooked pork.

YIELD
50 portions (2 pans)

PORTION SIZE
1 chop plus sauce

PAN SIZE
18 × 26-inch sheet pans
12 × 20 × 2-inch steam table pans

TEMPERATURE
375°F. Oven

DIETARY INFORMATION
May be used as written for general and no added salt diets. Diabetic diets — each serving provides 3 medium fat meat and 2 vegetable exchanges. Each serving provides 3 ounces cooked pork.

Barbecued Pork Chops

Refer to footnotes for special dietary information

INGREDIENTS	WEIGHTS/MEASURES	YIELD ADJUST.	METHOD
Pork chops	.17 pounds, 8 ounces (50 chops about 5 ounces each)		1. Put chops on lightly greased sheet pans; bake 1 hour; pour off as much fat as possible. 2. Put 25 chops, shingle style, in each of 2 steam table pans.

All-purpose flour . . . .
Salt . . . .
Pepper . . . .
Ground cloves . . . .
Worcestershire sauce . . . .
Salad mustard . . . .
Catsup . . . .
Finely chopped onions . . . .
Juice from spiced apples,
   spiced peaches or
   sweet pickles . . . .
	.1 cup
	.2 tablespoons
	.1 teaspoon
	.2 teaspoons
	.½ cup
	.½ cup
	.1½ quarts
	.1½ cups
	
	.1 quart
			3. Mix flour, salt, pepper and cloves; add Worcestershire sauce and mustard; mix well; add catsup, onions and juice; mix well; bring to a boil, stirring constantly.
			4. Pour half of the sauce over chops in each pan; cover lightly with aluminum foil; bake 1 hour and 15 minutes or until tender.

Baked Pork Chops with Dressing

Refer to footnotes for special dietary information

INGREDIENTS	WEIGHTS/MEASURES	YIELD ADJUST.	METHOD
Pork chops	17 pounds, 8 ounces (50 chops about 5 ounces each)		1. Put chops on lightly greased sheet pans; bake 1 hour; pour off as much fat as possible.
Dry bread, broken into pieces	2 pounds, 8 ounces.		2. Combine bread, margarine, onions, poultry seasoning and salt; mix lightly; add eggs and warm water and mix lightly.
Margarine, melted.	½ cup (4 ounces)		3. Put ¼ cup (No. 16 dipper) dressing on top of each chop.
Chopped onions	2¼ cups		
Poultry seasoning.	1 tablespoon		
Salt	1 teaspoon		
Slightly beaten eggs.	½ cup (about 3 medium)		
Warm water.	1½ quarts		
Water.	as necessary		4. Pour enough water in each pan to cover bottom of pan about ⅛ inch deep. 5. Bake 1 to 1½ hours or until chops are tender and dressing is lightly browned.

YIELD
50 portions (2 pans)

PORTION SIZE
1 chop plus dressing

PAN SIZE
18 × 26-inch sheet pans

TEMPERATURE
350°F. Oven

DIETARY INFORMATION
May be used as written for general, no added salt and bland diets. Diabetic diets — each serving provides 3½ medium fat meat and 1 bread exchanges. Each serving provides 3 ounces cooked pork.

YIELD
50 portions (2 pans)

PORTION SIZE
1 chop plus 2 tablespoons sauce

PAN SIZE
18 × 26-inch sheet pans
12 × 20 × 2-inch steam table pans

TEMPERATURE
350°F. Oven

VARIATION
Baked pork chops with tomato sauce:
Use cream of tomato soup instead of
cream of mushroom soup in step 3.

DIETARY INFORMATION
May be used as written for general, no
added salt, low fat, bland and restricted
residue diets. Diabetic diets — each
serving provides 3 medium fat meat and
1 vegetable exchanges. Each serving
provides 3 ounces cooked pork.

Baked Pork Chops with Mushroom Sauce

Refer to footnotes for special dietary information

INGREDIENTS	WEIGHTS/MEASURES	YIELD ADJUST.	METHOD
Pork chops	17 pounds, 8 ounces (50 chops about 5 ounces each)		1. Put chops on lightly greased sheet pans; bake 1 hour; pour off as much fat as possible. 2. Put 25 chops, shingle style, in each of 2 steam table pans.
Salt	2 tablespoons		
Nonfat dry milk	1 cup		3. Stir dry milk into hot water; add to soup; stir until smooth; pour ½ soup mixture over chops in each pan; cover pans tightly with aluminum foil; bake 1 hour or until chops are tender.
Hot water	3 cups		
Canned cream of mushroom soup	1 46-ounce can		

Spareribs with Barbecue Sauce

Refer to footnotes for special dietary information

INGREDIENTS	WEIGHTS/MEASURES	YIELD ADJUST.	METHOD
Pork spareribs	.37 pounds, 8 ounces (50 12-oz. portions)		1. Put ribs in pot; cover with water; bring to a boil; reduce heat; simmer 30 minutes.
Hot water	.to cover		2. Remove ribs from stock; put ribs in roasting pan. (Skim excess fat from stock; save stock to use with sauerkraut or for bean soup.
Barbecue Sauce:			3. Fry the onions and green peppers in butter or margarine until the onions are golden; add tomato puree, Worcestershire sauce, salt, pepper, vinegar and mustard; simmer, uncovered, 5 minutes.
Chopped onions	.1 cup		
Chopped fresh green peppers	.½ cup		
Margarine	.½ cup (4 ounces)		4. Pour barbecue sauce over ribs; cover and bake 1 hour. (Make sure sauce is well mixed in with spareribs.)
Tomato puree	.3 quarts (1 No. 10 can)		
Worcestershire sauce	.¼ cup		5. Uncover meat; bake another 30 minutes or until ribs are tender; baste frequently.
Salt	.2 tablespoons		
Pepper	.1 teaspoon		
Vinegar	.1 cup		
Salad mustard	.¼ cup		

YIELD
50 portions

PORTION SIZE
1 piece spareribs plus sauce

PAN SIZE
Heavy 5-gallon pot
Roasting pan

TEMPERATURE
350°F. Oven

NOTE
If desired, spareribs can be browned 30 minutes or until golden brown in 400°F. oven instead of being simmered in step 1. Pour off excess fat; continue to step 2.

DIETARY INFORMATION
May be used as written for general diets. Diabetic diets — each serving provides 3½ medium fat meat and 1 vegetable exchanges. Each serving provides 3 ounces cooked pork.

YIELD
50 portions

PORTION SIZE
1 piece spareribs plus ½ cup sauerkraut

PAN SIZE
Heavy 5-gallon pot
Roasting pan

TEMPERATURE
350°F. Oven

DIETARY INFORMATION
May be used as written for general diets. Diabetic diets — each serving provides 3½ medium fat meat exchanges. Each serving provides 3 ounces cooked pork.

Spareribs with Sauerkraut

Refer to footnotes for special dietary information

INGREDIENTS	WEIGHTS/MEASURES	YIELD ADJUST.	METHOD
Pork spareribs	.37 pounds, 8 ounces (50 12-oz. portions)		1. Put ribs in pot; cover with water; bring to a boil; reduce heat; simmer 30 minutes. 2. Remove ribs from stock; put ribs in roasting pan; sprinkle with salt and pepper. 3. Remove as much fat as possible from broth; pour 1 quart broth over spareribs; cover and bake 1 hour or until tender.
Hot water	.to cover		
Salt	.2 tablespoons		
Pepper.	.2 tablespoons		
Canned drained sauerkraut . . .	.1½ gallons (2 No. 10 cans)		4. Strain remaining broth; put strained broth back in pot with sauerkraut; cover and simmer until ribs are done. Drain the sauerkraut; serve hot with spareribs.

Sweet-Sour Spareribs

Refer to footnotes for special dietary information

INGREDIENTS	WEIGHTS/MEASURES	YIELD ADJUST.	METHOD
Pork spareribs	37 pounds, 8 ounces (50 12-oz portions)		1. Place spareribs in single layer, fat side up, in roasting pans; sprinkle with salt, pepper and garlic.
Salt	¼ cup		2. Bake 30 minutes at 400°F.; pour off excess fat; reduce heat to 350°F.; cook 20 minutes longer; pour off excess fat.
Pepper.	2 teaspoons		
Dehydrated garlic	1 tablespoon		
Brown sugar	1¼ cups		3. Dissolve sugar, cornstarch and ginger in water;; stir until smooth; add soy sauce and vinegar; cook, stirring frequently, until sauce thickens.
Cornstarch	1 cup		4. Add crushed pineapple with its juice to sauce; bring it to a boil; pour hot sauce over spareribs.
Ground ginger.	2 tablespoons		5. Bake 1½ hours or until meat is tender at 350°F.; baste occasionally with sauce. Skim fat off sauce before it is served.
Cold water.	2½ quarts		
Soy sauce	2 cups		
Vinegar	2 cups		
Canned crushed pineapple . . .	3 quarts (1 No. 10 can)		

YIELD
50 portions

PORTION SIZE
1 piece spareribs plus sauce

PAN SIZE
Roasting pan

TEMPERATURE
400°F. and 350°F. Oven

DIETARY INFORMATION
May be used as written for general diets. Diabetic diets — each serving provides 3½ medium fat meat and 1 bread exchanges. Each serving provides 3 ounces cooked pork.

YIELD
50 portions (about 2¼ gallons)

PORTION SIZE
¾ cup (6 ounces)

PAN SIZE
Heavy 5-gallon pot
Roasting pan

TEMPERATURE
350° F. Oven

DIETARY INFORMATION
May be used as written for general and no added salt diets. Diabetic diets — each serving provides 3 lean meat and 2 bread exchanges. Bland diets — omit fresh green peppers and pepper. Each serving provides 3 ounces of protein in the meat and beans.

Spanish-Style Lima Beans and Smoked Pork Shoulder

Refer to footnotes for special dietary information

INGREDIENTS	WEIGHTS/MEASURES	YIELD ADJUST.	METHOD
Dry lima beans . . . . .5 pounds (3 quarts) Water. .to cover			1. Look over beans; discard any dark ones; wash beans in cool water; drain and cover with cold water; bring to a boil; boil 2 minutes; cover and set off heat for 1 to 1½ hours.
Smoked pork shoulder . . . . . . .10 pounds Hot water . . . . .as necessary			2. Bone pork shoulder; cut meat into about 1-inch cubes; discard skin and any excess fat; add bone and cubed pork shoulder to beans; cover; simmer 1 hour; add water if necessary, to keep beans covered with water while they are cooking. 3. Remove bone from beans; discard bone; put beans in roasting pan. (Do not drain beans.)
Chopped celery. . . . . .1¼ quarts Chopped onions . . . . .1¼ quarts Chopped fresh 　green peppers. . . . . .1¼ quarts Thyme . . . . .2 teaspoons Pepper. . . . . .1 teaspoon Garlic granules . . . . .2 teaspoons			4. Add celery, onions, fresh green peppers, thyme, pepper and garlic granules to the beans and pork shoulder. Mix lightly but thoroughly. 5. Bake, uncovered, 30 to 45 minutes or until celery is tender.

Pork Cutlets with Cream Gravy

Refer to footnotes for special dietary information

INGREDIENTS	WEIGHTS/MEASURES	YIELD ADJUST.	METHOD
Pork cutlets................	12 pounds, 8 ounces (50 4-oz. cutlets)		1. Beat eggs, water, salt and pepper together with a wire whisk or hand beater. Dip cutlets in egg mixture; dredge in bread crumbs; place on lightly greased sheet pans; bake about 1¼ hours or until browned and tender.
Eggs	2 cups (10 to 12 medium)		
Cold water................	¾ cup		
Salt.....................	2 tablespoons		
Pepper...................	1 teaspoon		
Dry bread crumbs..........	1 pounds (1 quart)		
Hot water	1 quart		2. Remove baked cutlets to serving pans; rinse sheet pans with hot water; scrape brown bits off pans and put with hot water into a saucepan; add milk. Add flour, salt and pepper to cold water; stir to form a smooth paste. Pour flour mixture into milk mixture; cook and stir over moderate heat until smooth and thickened and the starchy taste is gone. Serve the hot gravy with the hot cutlets.
Milk......................	2¼ quarts		
All-purpose flour...........	1 cup		
Salt	2 teaspoons		
Pepper...................	½ teaspoon		
Cold water................	2 cups		

YIELD
50 portions

PORTION SIZE
1 cutlet plus
¼ cup (2-ounce ladle) gravy

PAN SIZE
18 × 26-inch sheet pans

TEMPERATURE
350°F. Oven

DIETARY INFORMATION
May be used as written for general and no added salt diets. Diabetic diets — each serving provides 3 lean meat and 1 lowfat milk exchanges. Bland diets — omit pepper. Each serving provides 3 ounces cooked pork.

YIELD
50 portions (about 2¼ gallons)

PORTION SIZE
¾ cup (6-ounce ladle)

PAN SIZE
Roasting pan
Heavy 5-gallon pot

TEMPERATURE
350°F. Oven

NOTE
Diced raw beef may be substituted for up to 50% of the pork in step 1.

DIETARY INFORMATION
May be used as written for general, no added salt and low cholesterol diets. Diabetic diets — each serving provides 3 medium fat meat and 2 vegetable exchanges. Bland diets — omit pepper. Each serving provides 3 ounces cooked pork.

Chop Suey

Refer to footnotes for special dietary information

INGREDIENTS	WEIGHTS/MEASURES	YIELD ADJUST.	METHOD
Boneless pork shoulder, cut in 1-inch cubes ....14 pounds Salt ....3 tablespoons Pepper....................1 teaspoon			1. Put pork in roasting pan; sprinkle with salt and pepper; bake, uncovered, about 45 minutes to 1 hour or until browned; stirring occasionally. Put meat in a colander and drain off fat; put drained meat in pot.
Water....................3 quarts Soy sauce ....1½ cups Bead molasses............7 tablespoons			2. Add water, soy sauce and molasses to pork; bring to a boil; reduce heat; simmer, covered, about 45 minutes or until meat is tender; skim off any fat which rises to the top.
Sliced onions ....1 gallon Celery, cut in ¼-inch pieces...........1 gallon			3. Add onions and celery to pork; cover and simmer 20 mins.
Canned bean sprouts ....3 quarts (1 No. 10 can) Cornstarch ....1½ cups			4. Drain bean sprouts; combine liquid from bean sprouts with cornstarch; stir to form a smooth paste; add the smooth paste slowly to hot meat mixture, stirring constantly; cook 8 to 10 minutes or until thickened. 5. Add bean sprouts; mix well; reheat to a simmer and serve hot over rice or fried noodles.

Pork and Vegetable Stew

Refer to footnotes for special dietary information

INGREDIENTS	WEIGHTS/MEASURES	YIELD ADJUST.	METHOD
Boneless pork shoulder, cut in 1-inch cubes . . . . .14 pounds Salt . . . . .2 tablespoons Pepper. . . . . .1 teaspoon Chopped onions . . . . .1 quart Ground allspice. . . . . .1 tablespoon Garlic granules . . . . .2 teaspoons			1. Put pork in roasting pan; sprinkle with salt, pepper, onions, allspice and garlic; bake, uncovered, about 1 hour or until browned; stirring occasionally. Put meat in a colander and drain off fat; return meat to roasting pan; put pan on top of range.
Hot water . . . . .1 gallon			2. Pour hot water over meat; bring to a boil; reduce heat; simmer, covered, about 45 minutes or until meat is tender.
Canned mixed vegetables . . . .3 quarts (1 No. 10 can) Canned peas. . . . . .3 quarts (1 No. 10 can) Cooked diced potatoes. . . . . .2 quarts			3. Drain vegetables well; keep vegetable juice for later use. 4. Add vegetables and 2 quarts of their liquid to meat; reheat to a simmer.
All-purpose flour . . . . .1 cup Salt . . . . .1 tablespoon Pepper. . . . . .½ teaspoon Cold water. . . . . .2 cups			5. Combine flour, salt, pepper and cold water; stir to form a smooth paste. Add paste to simmering stew; stir gently until thickened. Use a little of the vegetable juice from step 3 to thin gravy, if necessary. Serve hot.

YIELD
50 portions (about 3¼ gallons)

PORTION SIZE
1 cup (8-ounce ladle)

PAN SIZE
Roasting pan

TEMPERATURE
350°F. Oven

DIETARY INFORMATION
May be used as written for general and no added salt diets. Diabetic diets — each serving provides 3½ lean meat and 1 bread exchanges. Bland diets — omit pepper. Each serving provides 3 ounces cooked pork.

YIELD
50 portions (about 3¼ gallons)

PORTION SIZE
1 cup (8-ounce ladle)

PAN SIZE
Roasting pan

TEMPERATURE
350°F. Oven

DIETARY INFORMATION
May be used as written for general, bland, no added salt and low cholesterol diets. Diabetic diets — each serving provides 3 medium fat meat and 1½ bread exchanges. Each serving provides 3 ounces cooked pork.

Pork and Sweet Potato Stew

Refer to footnotes for special dietary information

INGREDIENTS	WEIGHTS/MEASURES	YIELD ADJUST.	METHOD
Boneless pork shoulder, cut in 1-inch cubes . . . . .14 pounds Cornstarch . . . . .1 cup Chopped onions . . . . .1 quart			1. Put pork in roasting pan; sprinkle with cornstarch; stir to mix well; sprinkle with onions; bake, uncovered, about 1 hour or until browned; stirring occasionally. Put meat in a colander; drain off fat; return meat to roasting pan; put pan on top of range.
Canned sweet potatoes or yams . . . . .1½ gallons (2 No. 10 cans)			2. Drain sweet potatoes or yams; reserve 1 quart juice for use in step 3; cut sweet potatoes into pieces about the size of an eighth of a potato.
Water. . . . . .1½ quarts Ground ginger. . . . . .2 tablespoons Soy sauce . . . . .1 cup Salt .2 teaspoons			3. Combine 1 quart juice from sweet potatoes or yams, water, ginger, soy sauce and salt; mix well; add to the meat, bring to a boil; reduce heat, cover and simmer 45 minutes or until meat is tender. 4. Add sweet potatoes or yams to meat; reheat over low heat; serve hot.

Pork au Gratin

Refer to footnotes for special dietary information

INGREDIENTS	WEIGHTS/MEASURES	YIELD ADJUST.	METHOD
Lean ground pork . . . . .9 pounds, 8 ounces Chopped onions . . . . .1½ quarts			1. Put pork in roasting pan; sprinkle onions over pork; bake, uncovered, about 1 hour or until browned; stirring occasionally. Put meat in a colander; drain off fat; return meat to pan.
Shell macaroni . . . . .2 pounds (2 quarts) Hot water . . . . .2 gallons Vegetable oil . . . . .2 tablespoons			2. Stir macaroni into hot water; mix lightly; add vegetable oil; cook about 6 minutes or until barely tender; drain well.
Sage . . . . .2 tablespoons Catsup . . . . .1½ cups Salt . . . . .2 tablespoons Pepper. . . . . .1 teaspoon Chopped pimiento . . . . .½ cup Condensed cream of celery soup . . . . .2 46-ounce cans			3. Combine sage, catsup, salt, pepper, pimiento and soup; mix well; add to meat mixture.
Boiling water. . . . . .1½ quarts			4. Stir water and shell macaroni into meat mixture; mix lightly; cover tightly; bake 30 minutes.
Grated or ground cheddar cheese . . . . .1 pound, 8 ounces			5. Remove cover; sprinkle with cheese; return to oven; bake uncovered, 15 minutes, or until cheese is melted.

YIELD
50 portions (about 3¼ gallons)

PORTION SIZE
1 cup (8 ounces)

PAN SIZE
Roasting pan
Heavy 5-gallon pot

TEMPERATURE
375°F. Oven

DIETARY INFORMATION
May be used as written for general and no added salt diets. Diabetic diets — each serving provides 3 lean meat, 1 bread and 1 vegetable exchanges. Bland diets — omit pepper. Each serving provides 3 ounces cooked pork.

YIELD
50 portions (about 3¼ gallons)

PORTION SIZE
1 cup (8 ounces)

PAN SIZE
Roasting pan

TEMPERATURE
375°F. Oven

DIETARY INFORMATION
May be used as written for general, no added salt, bland and low cholesterol diets. Diabetic diets — each serving provides 3 medium fat meat, 1 bread and 1 vegetable exchanges. Each serving provides 3 ounces cooked pork.

Pork with Rice

Refer to footnotes for special dietary information

INGREDIENTS	WEIGHTS/MEASURES	YIELD ADJUST.	METHOD
Pork shoulder, cut in 1-inch cubes . . . . .14 pounds Chopped onions . . . . 1½ quarts			1. Put pork in roasting pan; sprinkle with onions; bake, uncovered, about 1 hour or until browned; stirring occasionally. Put meat in a colander; drain off fat; put drained meat in roasting pan.
Hot chicken stock. . . . . .1 gallon Chopped celery. . . . . .1 quart Long grain rice . . . . .3 pounds (6¾ cups) Soy sauce . . . . .1½ cups			2. Add chicken stock, celery, rice, and soy sauce to meat; mix lightly but thoroughly. 3. Cover tightly; bake 1 hour and 15 minutes or until pork and rice are tender.
Chopped pimiento . . . . .1 cup			4. Fold pimiento into pork and rice mixture; serve hot.

Sweet-Sour Pork

Refer to footnotes for special dietary information

INGREDIENTS	WEIGHTS/MEASURES	YIELD ADJUST.	METHOD
Boneless pork shoulder, cut in 1-inch cubes . . . . .14 pounds			1. Put pork in roasting pan; bake, uncovered about 45 minutes to 1 hour or until browned, stirring occasionally; put meat in a colander; drain off fat; put meat in pot.
Chicken broth . . . . .2 quarts			2. Add chicken broth to pork; bring to a boil; reduce heat; simmer, covered, about 45 minutes or until meat is tender; skim off any fat which rises to top.
Brown sugar . . . . .2 cups Cornstarch . . . . .1 cup Pineapple juice . . . . .3 cups Vinegar . . . . .2 cups Soy sauce . . . . .1½ cups Salt . . . . .2 teaspoons			3. Combine sugar, cornstarch, juice, vinegar, soy sauce and salt; mix until smooth; add to meat mixture; cook and stir over low heat until thickened.
Julienne-cut fresh green peppers . . . . .1 quart Coarsely chopped onions. . . . .1½ quarts			4. Add fresh green peppers and onions to meat; cook 15 minutes over low heat; stirring frequently.
Medium size tomatoes cut in eighths . . . . .3 pounds Drained pineapple chunks . . . .3 quarts (1 No. 10 can)			5. Add tomatoes and pineapple to meat mixture; heat gently, stirring as little as possible; serve hot over rice or fried noodles.

YIELD
50 portions (about 2¼ gallons)

PORTION SIZE
¾ cup (6-ounce ladle)

PAN SIZE
Roasting pan
Heavy 5-gallon pot

TEMPERATURE
350°F. Oven

NOTE
This recipe should be prepared as closely as possible to serving time. Steps 1 and 2 may be prepared earlier and refrigerated but remaining steps must be prepared at the last minute.

DIETARY INFORMATION
May be used as written for general, no added salt and low cholesterol diets.

YIELD
50 portions

PORTION SIZE
3 ounces

PAN SIZE
Roasting pan

TEMPERATURE
325°F. Oven

NOTE
If frozen roasts are used, they should be cooked as follows:
Rolled leg: 4 to 5 hours.
Rolled shoulder: 3½ to 4¼ hours.

DIETARY INFORMATION
May be used as written for general, low cholesterol, low fat, and no added salt diets. Diabetic diets — each serving provides 3 meat exchanges. Bland diets — omit pepper. Restricted residue diets — omit pepper and garlic. Each serving provides 3 ounces cooked lamb.

Roast Lamb

Refer to footnotes for special dietary information

INGREDIENTS	WEIGHTS/MEASURES	YIELD ADJUST.	METHOD
Boneless lamb roast (rolled leg or shoulder) . . . . .13 pounds, 8 ounces Salt . . . . .2 tablespoons Pepper . . . . .1½ teaspoons Finely chopped garlic . . . . .3 cloves			1. Rub outside of roasts with salt, pepper and garlic. 2. Put roasts fat side up in roasting pan without crowding, do not cover pan or add water. 3. Insert a meat thermometer in thickest part of meat; cook until meat thermometer registers 180°F. or Cook rolled leg 3 to 4 hours. Cook rolled shoulder 2¼ to 3¼ hours, depending upon size of roasts. 4. Remove meat from pan; cool 20 minutes before it is sliced. (If the meat is not to be used right away, it should be refrigerated after it has cooled for 30 minutes.) 5. Use any drippings for making gravy. If gravy is not to be made for that meal, drippings should be refrigerated until used. (Scrape the brown particles from pan and use with drippings for gravy.)

Lamb Stew

Refer to footnotes for special dietary information

INGREDIENTS	WEIGHTS/MEASURES	YIELD ADJUST.	METHOD
Boneless lamb stew meat . . . . 14 pounds, 8 ounces Minced garlic . . . . 3 cloves Salt . . . . 2 tablespoons Pepper. . . . . 1 teaspoon Chopped onions . . . . 1 cup			1. Put lamb in roasting pan; do not add any shortening or other fat; sprinkle garlic, salt, pepper and onions over the meat. Roast, uncovered, about 1 hour or until meat is browned; drain off as much fat as possible.
Hot water . . . . 1 gallon			2. Pour hot water over meat; cover pan and continue to bake about 2 hours or until meat is tender.

Carrots, cut in
   1-inch cubes . . . . 3 quarts
Potatoes, cut in
   1-inch cubes . . . . 3 quarts
Coarsely chopped onions. . . . . 2 quarts
Salt . . . . 2 tablespoons
Hot water . . . . as necessary
			3. Cover vegetables with hot water; add salt; bring to a boil; cover and cook about 20 minutes or until tender. Drain vegetables but save liquid to use for gravy.

All-purpose flour . . . . 1½ cups Cold water. . . . . 1 quart			4. Remove cover of roaster after meat is tender; put roaster and meat on top of range. 5. Combine flour and water; mix until smooth; add to meat and juice, stirring constantly to prevent lumping. Add as much of the vegetable water as necessary to give you a medium thick gravy.
Drained, canned green beans . . . . 3 quarts (1 No. 10 can)			6. Add the green beans and the cooked vegetables to the meat and gravy. Add more salt, if necessary. Serve hot.

YIELD
50 portions (about 3¼ gallons)

PORTION SIZE
1 cup (8-ounce ladle)

PAN SIZE
Roasting pan

TEMPERATURE
375°F. Oven

DIETARY INFORMATION
May be used as written for general, low cholesterol, and no added salt diets.
Diabetic diets — each serving provides 3 lean meat and 1 bread exchanges.
Bland diets — omit pepper. Each serving provides 3 ounces cooked lamb.

Chapter 5
Poultry

Information 106

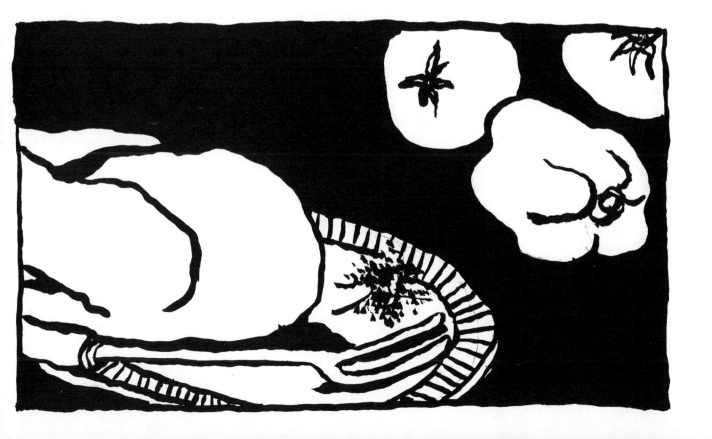

Poultry Information

General

All poultry is highly perishable and extreme care should be taken to keep it clean and pure at all times.

Precooked, diced or sliced chicken or turkey have been used in various recipes in this book because of their economy and labor saving qualities.

Never refreeze poultry once it has been defrosted. However, if there is any leftover, cooked poultry, it should be well wrapped in freezer paper or aluminum foil and frozen for use in a la kings or for ground, chopped or pureed poultry. It should be labeled, frozen at 0°F. and used within a month.

Defrost poultry by putting it in the refrigerator for 24 to 72 hours. Plan defrosting so that it can be used as soon as possible after it is defrosted. See information on turkey for special instructions for defrosting turkeys.

Chicken

Fresh chicken should be used whenever possible. Fresh chicken should be packed in ice when delivered and should not be kept over 1 day.

Chickens are marketed younger now than formerly and yield more meat in relation to bone. They are available fresh, quick frozen or deep chilled.

Ready-to-cook chicken is available whole, split, quartered or in parts. Recipes in this book specify the type of chicken to be purchased and the amounts necessary to serve 50 persons.

Turkey

Turkey has become a popular menu item because of its economy and high yield of cooked meat. Tests have shown that the large institutional size turkeys (20 to 30 pounds) are more economical because they yield a higher percentage of cooked weight and because they require less labor for a given number of portions. The Broad Breasted Bronze or Broad Breasted White turkeys give a particularly high yield of cooked turkey with a higher percentage of white meat.

Turkeys may also be purchased in parts like chicken or in boneless, cooked or raw, turkey rolls.

It is recommended that turkeys for institutional use be roasted without stuffing and all directions in this book are for unstuffed turkeys. The quantity of dressing needed is usually greater than the capacity of the turkey and the quality of the meat and dressing is just as good, if not better, if the stuffing is cooked separately. There is danger of food poisoning if the stuffing is not thoroughly baked, and the danger is less if the stuffing is in a pan instead of in the turkey. Stuffing baked in pans is also easier to serve than stuffing baked in the turkey. It is particularly important for some special diets that the stuffing be baked separately so that it won't absorb any of the fat from the turkey.

Almost all of the turkeys on the market today are eviscerated, ready-to-cook birds. They have been efficiently processed in modern sanitary plants and they have probably been packed in plastic bags. They should be defrosted by keeping the bird in its plastic bag in the refrigerator for 24 to 72 hours or they may be defrosted, still in the bag, under running cold water for 4 to 6 hours. Be sure never to use warm water when defrosting turkeys because this will break down the tissue of the meat and may cause spoilage of the meat.

The giblets of the turkeys are wrapped in parchment paper inside the neck cavity. Be sure to remove them before the bird is cooked.

The turkey should be washed lightly and drained thoroughly before it is used.

Roast Turkey

Refer to footnotes for special dietary information

INGREDIENTS	WEIGHTS/MEASURES	YIELD ADJUST.	METHOD
Ready-to-cook turkey	21 pounds, 8 ounces		1. Wash thawed turkey inside and outside with cool running water; drain thoroughly; pat dry with clean cloth or paper towels.
Salt . . . . Pepper	as necessary ½ teaspoon		2. Rub inside cavity of turkey with salt and pepper.
Vegetable oil	¼ cup		3. Brush skin of turkey with oil using a pastry brush. 4. Place turkey breast side up in roasting pan. Do not crowd turkey; do not cover pan or add water to pan. 5. Insert a meat thermometer in center of inside muscle of thigh; cook to an interior temperature of 185°F. or until the drumstick joint can be moved up and down easily and the breast feels soft. Baste turkey every half hour with drippings. If turkey begins to get too brown, cover with a loose tent made of aluminum foil.

or

SIZE	TIME
6 to 8 pounds	2 to 2½ hours
8 to 12 pounds	2½ to 3 hours
12 to 16 pounds	3 to 3¾ hours
16 to 20 pounds	3¾ to 4½ hours
20 to 24 pounds	4½ to 5½ hours

6. Cool cooked turkey 20 minutes; slice and serve hot.

or

Cool turkey on a rack until cool enough to handle. Remove meat from bones; spread pieces of meat in a clean pan to cool but do not make meat more than 1 layer thick in pan. As soon as turkey is cool, wrap loosely in wax paper or aluminum foil and refrigerate until used but not more than 2 days.

7. Turkey may be reheated by covering it with a damp cloth and heating it in a moderate (350°F.) oven 30 minutes to 1 hour depending upon the quantity of turkey in pan.

YIELD
50 portions

PORTION SIZE
3 ounces

PAN SIZE
Roasting pan

TEMPERATURE
325°F. Oven

NOTES
1. Turkeys must be completely thawed before they are cooked. THEY SHOULD NOT BE THAWED IN THE KITCHEN. They should be thawed in refrigerator. A large turkey will take 2 or 3 days to thaw and a smaller turkey will take about 1 to 2 days to thaw.
2. Dressing should be cooked separately in a separate pan.
3. NEVER partially cook a turkey 1 day and finish cooking it the next.
4. Always refrigerate leftover turkey and dressing as soon as possible.
5. If you intend to use leftover turkey more than 2 days later, it should be wrapped in aluminum foil and frozen.

DIETARY INFORMATION
May be used as written for general, low fat, low cholesterol, no added salt and soft diets. Diabetic diets — each serving provides 3 lean meat exchanges. Bland and restricted residue diets — omit pepper. Skin must be removed for low fat and low cholesterol diets. Each serving provides 3 ounces cooked turkey.

Roast Boneless Raw Turkey Rolls

Refer to footnotes for special dietary information

YIELD
50 Portions

PORTION SIZE
3 ounces

PAN SIZE
Roasting pan

TEMPERATURE
350°F. Oven

VARIATION
Roast boneless cooked turkey rolls:
Slice thawed turkey in 1-ounce slices.
Lay slices in a steam table pan with
slices overlapping; cover with aluminum
foil. Refrigerate until ready to use but do
not slice more than 12 hours before it is
used. Add 2 cups boiling hot chicken
stock to each steam table pan; cover
and heat to a simmer but do not cook.

DIETARY INFORMATION
May be used as written for general, low
fat, low cholesterol, bland, no added
salt, soft and restricted residue diets.
Diabetic diets — each serving provides
3 lean meat exchanges. Each serving
provides 3 ounces of cooked turkey.

INGREDIENTS	WEIGHTS/MEASURES	YIELD ADJUST.	METHOD
Thawed boneless raw turkey roll	15 pounds, 8 ounces		1. Remove any casings and put turkey rolls in roasting pan; brush with melted margarine. Put meat thermometer in center of one of the turkey rolls.
Margarine, melted	as necessary		2. Roast, uncovered, 3½ to 4 hours or until meat thermometer registers an internal temperature of 175°F.
			3. Remove turkey rolls from oven; let stand 30 minutes to absorb juices and for best results in slicing.
			4. Remove strings and skin; slice turkey with a sharp knife; cover with skin until turkey is served. Save juices for gravy or stock.

Roast Chicken

Refer to footnotes for special dietary information

INGREDIENTS	WEIGHTS/MEASURES	YIELD ADJUST.	METHOD
2 to 2½ pound broiler-fryers cut in quarters. . . . . .50 quarters or (about 30 pounds) Legs and thighs . . . . .50 pieces or (about 20 pounds) ½ breasts . . . . .50 pieces (about 17 pounds, 8 oz.) Salt . . . . .2 tablespoons Pepper. . . . . .1 teaspoon Hot water or chicken stock. . . .as necessary			1. Wash chicken well under running water; drain well. 2. Put pieces or quarters of chicken, skin side up, on lightly greased sheet pans; do not crowd pieces of chicken. 3. Sprinkle pieces with salt and pepper. 4. Bake 1 hour or until lightly browned. Take pieces of chicken from the sheet pans and put in a roasting pan (do not pile them over 2 layers deep). Add about ¼ inch of hot water or chicken stock to bottom of roaster; cover tightly and cook another ½ hour or until tender.

YIELD
50 portions

PORTION SIZE
¼ chicken or 1 leg with thigh or ½ breast

PAN SIZE
18 × 26-inch sheet pans
Roasting pan

TEMPERATURE
350°F. Oven

VARIATION
Barbecued chicken: Brush chicken with a mild barbecue sauce after it is put into roasting pan. Cover pan and continue to cook another half hour or until tender. Brush chicken again with sauce if it seems to be getting dry. Do not add hot water or chicken stock to pan in step 5.

DIETARY INFORMATION
May be used as written for general, soft, no added salt, bland and restricted residue diets. Bland and restricted residue diets — omit pepper. Low fat diets — remove skin before baking. Diabetic diets — each serving provides 3 lean meat exchanges. Low fat diets — remove skin before baking and do not add any fat from the sheet pans along with the chicken in the roaster. Diabetic diets—each serving provides 3 lean meat exchanges. Each serving provides 3 ounces cooked chicken.

YIELD
50 portions

PORTION SIZE
¼ chicken (2 pieces)

PAN SIZE
Roasting pan

TEMPERATURE
350°F. Oven

DIETARY INFORMATION
May be used as written for general, no added salt and bland diets. Diabetic diets — each serving provides 4 lean meat exchanges. Each serving provides 3 ounces cooked chicken.

Savory Baked Chicken

Refer to footnotes for special dietary information

INGREDIENTS	WEIGHTS/MEASURES	YIELD ADJUST.	METHOD
2 to 2½ pound broiler-fryers cut into 8 pieces . . . . 28 pounds			1. Wash chicken thoroughly under running water. Drain well; put chicken in a roasting pan.
Salt . . . . .2 tablespoons Vegetable oil . . . . .1 cup Celery salt. . . . . .1 tablespoon Garlic salt . . . . .1 tablespoon Worcestershire sauce. . . . . . . .½ cup Soy sauce . . . . .¾ cup			2. Combine salt, oil, celery salt, garlic salt, Worcestershire sauce and soy sauce; mix well; pour over chicken. Refrigerate chicken and seasonings in refrigerator for 1 to 3 hours, turning chicken in the sauce every half hour. 3. Bake chicken and sauce 1½ to 2 hours or until tender, basting chicken about every half hour with the sauce in the pan.

Cornflake Crumb Chicken

Refer to footnotes for special dietary information

INGREDIENTS	WEIGHTS/MEASURES	YIELD ADJUST.	METHOD
2 to 2½ pound broiler-fryers cut into 8 pieces . . . . .28 pounds Milk . . . . .1 quart			1. Wash chicken well under running water; drain well; pat dry with clean cloths or paper towels. 2. Dip each piece of chicken in milk.
Cornflake crumbs . . . . .2½ quarts Salt . . . . .¼ cup Paprika . . . . .1 tablespoon Pepper. . . . . .1 teaspoon			3. Mix cornflake crumbs, salt, paprika and pepper together; put in a shallow pan. 4. Dredge chicken in seasoned crumbs; put on well-greased sheet pans; be careful not to crowd the chicken. 5. Bake chicken 1½ hours or until tender.

YIELD
50 portions (2 pans)

PORTION SIZE
2 pieces

PAN SIZE
18 × 26-inch sheet pans

TEMPERATURE
350°F.

DIETARY INFORMATION
May be used as written for general, low fat, low cholesterol, soft and no added salt diets. Diabetic diets — each serving provides 3 lean meat and ½ bread exchanges. Bland diets — omit pepper. Each serving provides 3 ounces cooked chicken.

YIELD
50 portions

PORTION SIZE
2 pieces

PAN SIZE
18 × 26-inch sheet pans
Roaster
8-quart pot

TEMPERATURE
350°F. Oven

DIETARY INFORMATION
May be used as written for general and no added salt diets. Diabetic diets — each serving provides 4 lean meat and 1/2 vegetable exchanges. Bland diets — omit pepper. Each serving provides 3 ounces of cooked chicken.

Chicken Fricassee

Refer to footnotes for special dietary information

INGREDIENTS	WEIGHTS/MEASURES	YIELD ADJUST.	METHOD
2 to 2½ pound broiler-fryers cut into 8 pieces . . . . .28 pounds			1. Wash chicken thoroughly under running cool water. Drain well. Pat dry with a clean cloth or paper towels. Place chicken pieces with skin side up on lightly greased sheet pans. Bake 1 to 1½ hours or until browned. Place hot chicken in roaster. Discard fat and liquid.
Chopped onions . . . . .2 quarts Chopped carrots. . . . . .1 quart Chopped celery. . . . . .1 cup			2. Scatter onions, carrots and celery over chicken pieces.
Vegetable oil . . . . .½ cup All-purpose flour . . . . .1½ cups Cool fat-free chicken broth . . . .1 gallon Salt . . . . .2 tablespoons Pepper (optional). . . . . .½ teaspoon Thyme. . . . . .2 teaspoons			3. Place oil and flour in heavy pot and cook and stir over medium heat until mixture is smooth and lightly browned. Add broth, salt, pepper and thyme and cook and stir until thickened. 4. Pour the hot sauce over the hot chicken. Stir lightly to distribute the sauce. 5. Cover tightly and bake 1 hour. Remove cover and bake another 30 minute or until the chicken is very tender. Serve chicken hot with some of the sauce over noodles or rice.

Baked Chicken or Turkey and Noodles

Refer to footnotes for special dietary information

YIELD
50 portions (1 pan)

PORTION SIZE
3/4 cup (6 ounces)

PAN SIZE
Heavy 5-gallon pot
Roasting pan

TEMPERATURE
350°F. Oven

INGREDIENTS	WEIGHTS/MEASURES	YIELD ADJUST.	METHOD
Egg noodles . . . . .3 pounds Boiling water. . . . . .3 gallons Salt . . . . .3 tablespoons Vegetable oil . . . . .2 tablespoons			1. Add noodles to boiling salted water; add oil and cook, stirring occasionally, 15 minutes or until tender. Drain well but do not rinse noodles.
Chicken fat or margarine, melted. . . . . .1 cup All-purpose flour . . . . .3 cups White pepper. . . . . .1 teaspoon Hot chicken stock. . . . . .1½ gallons Salt . . . . .as necessary			2. Combine fat and flour; add pepper and mix until smooth; add to hot stock; cook and stir over low heat until thickened and smooth and the starchy taste is gone. (If chicken stock is not available, prepare with hot water and chicken soup and gravy base.) Taste; add salt if necessary.

Precooked diced chicken or
   turkey with skin and gristle
   removed . . . . .6 pounds,
                  4 ounces
Paprika . . . . .1 tablespoon
			3. Combine noodles, sauce and chicken or turkey; mix lightly and put into well-greased roasting pan.
			4. Sprinkle top lightly with paprika; bake 30 minutes; serve hot.

NOTES
1. 9 pounds, 8 ounces of chicken or turkey may be used in step 3 instead of the 6 pounds, 4 ounces chicken or turkey. If 9 pounds, 8 ounces of chicken or turkey are used, each portion will provide 3 ounces of cooked chicken or turkey.
2. Chicken or turkey and noodles may be served without baking if desired.
3. 3 pounds macaroni may be used instead of 3 pounds of egg noodles in step 1, if desired.

DIETARY INFORMATION
May be used as written for general, low fat and no added salt diets. Diabetic diets — each serving provides 3 lean meat and 1½ bread exchanges. Bland and restricted residue diets — omit pepper. Low cholesterol diets — remove all skin and fat from chicken or turkey and use margarine in step 2. Each serving provides 2 ounces cooked chicken or turkey.

YIELD
50 portions (about 2¼ gallons)

PORTION SIZE
¾ cup (6-ounce ladle)

PAN SIZE
Heavy 5-gallon pot

DIETARY INFORMATION
May be used as written for general, bland, low fat, low cholesterol and no added salt diets. Diabetic diets — each serving provides 2 lean meat and 1 vegetable exchanges. Each serving provides 2 ounces cooked chicken or turkey.

Chicken or Turkey Chop Suey

Refer to footnotes for special dietary information

INGREDIENTS WEIGHTS/MEASURES	YIELD ADJUST.	METHOD
Cornstarch . . . . .1½ cups Cold water. . . . . .1 gallon Soy sauce . . . . .1½ cups Salt . . . . .1 tablespoon Sugar. . . . . .½ cup Chicken soup and gravy base. .½ cup Celery, cut into ½-inch pieces .3 quarts Sliced onions . . . . .1½ quarts		1. Mix cornstarch with 3 cups water to form a smooth mixture. Add soy sauce, salt, sugar and soup and gravy base along with the cornstarch mixture to the remaining cold water in the pot. Stir well. 2. Add celery and onions to mixture in the pot, bring to a boil, reduce heat and simmer 20 minutes, stirring frequently.
Canned, drained bean sprouts .3 quarts (1 No. 10 can)		3. Add bean sprouts to vegetable mixture. Bring to a boil. Reduce heat and simmer another 2 minutes.

Precooked diced chicken or
   turkey with gristle, fat and
   skin removed. . . . . .6 pounds,
4 ounces
		4. Add chicken or turkey to vegetable mixture. Mix well, reheat and serve hot over rice.

Creamy Chicken Lasagna

Refer to footnotes for special dietary information

INGREDIENTS	WEIGHTS/MEASURES	YIELD ADJUST.	METHOD
Ricotta cheese . . . . .4 pounds Eggs . . . . .3 cups (15 to 18 medium) Grated Parmesan cheese . . . . .1 cup Chopped parsley. . . . . .¼ cup Garlic powder . . . . .1 tablespoon			1. Combine ricotta cheese, eggs, Parmesan cheese, parsley and garlic powder in mixer bowl. Mix at low speed to blend but do not whip. Set aside for later use. If it is to be used more than 1 hour later, the mixture should be refrigerated. However, it should be returned to room temperature before it is used.
Hot water . . . . .3½ gallons Salt . . . . .2 tablespoons Vegetable oil . . . . .2 tablespoons Lasagna noodles . . . . .3 pounds, 8 ounces			2. Place water, salt and oil in pot. Bring to a boil; add noodles and cook according to directions on the package or until tender. Drain noodles well as soon as they are cooked. Noodles may be allowed to stand in cold water until needed, if they are cooked before the lasagna is assembled.
Canned mushroom slices and pieces . . . . .2 1-pound cans Water. . . . . .as necessary Chicken soup and gravy base. .¼ cup Canned cream of chicken soup 2 46-oz. cans Cubed cooked chicken with fat and gristle removed . . . . . . .3 pounds			3. Drain mushrooms well. Set mushrooms aside. Add water to mushroom juice to total 1½ quarts liquid. Dissolve soup and gravy base in liquid and mix with the soup. 4. Add reserved mushrooms to the soup mixture. Mix lightly and use for assembling lasagna.

Continues on next page

YIELD
48 portions (2 pans)

PORTION SIZE
1 square

PAN SIZE
12 x 20 × 2-inch steam table pans
5-gallon pot

TEMPERATURE
350°F. Oven

VARIATION
Creamy vegetable lasagna: Delete chicken and chicken soup. Substitute 2 46-ounce cans of cream of mushroom soup combined with 2½ quarts of cooked chopped drained vegetables such as carrots, broccoli, cauliflower, green or yellow wax beans or peas.

DIETARY INFORMATION
May be used as written for general, bland, no added salt and mechanical soft diets. Diabetic diets — each serving provides 2 bread and 3 medium fat meat exchanges. Each serving provides 3 ounces cooked chicken and cheese.

Continued from preceding page

INGREDIENTS	WEIGHTS/MEASURES	YIELD ADJUST.	METHOD

Coarsely grated mozzarella . . .3 pounds
Grated Parmesan cheese . . . . .⅔ cup
Leaf oregano. . . . . .2 tablespoons
			5. Assembling instructions for lasagna: (each pan)
			    1. 3 cups mushroom sauce in the bottom of each of 2 pans.
			    2. ⅙ of the noodles placed flat and in rows on top of the mushroom chicken sauce.
			    3. 3 cups cheese filling.
			    4. 12 ounces mozzarella cheese.
			    5. 3 cups mushroom chicken sauce.
			    6. ⅙ of the noodles placed flat and in rows.
			    7. 3 cups cheese filling.
			    8. 12 ounces mozzarella cheese.
			    9. 3 cups mushroom chicken sauce.
			    10. ⅙ of the noodles placed flat and in rows.
			    11. 3 cups of the mushroom chicken sauce.
			    12. ⅓ cup Parmesan cheese.
			    13. Sprinkle with 1 tablespoon oregano.
			6. Bake about 1 hour or until the top is bubbling and lightly browned.
			7. Let stand about 20 minutes at room temperature to firm up before cutting each pan 4 × 6. Serve hot.

Turkey Loaf

Refer to footnotes for special dietary information

INGREDIENTS	WEIGHTS/MEASURES	YIELD ADJUST.	METHOD
Ground, raw, boneless turkey . .11 pounds Eggs .2 cups (10-12 medium) Chicken soup and gravy base. .1/2 cup Poultry seasoning. . . . . .1 tablespoon Salt .1 tablespoon Finely chopped onions . . . . . . .1 cup Dry bread crumbs . . . . .5 cups (1¼ quarts)			1. Combine raw turkey, eggs, soup and gravy base, poultry seasoning, salt, onions and bread crumbs in a mixer bowl. Mix 2 minutes at medium speed or until well blended; do not overmix. 2. Spread turkey in loaf pans to about 1 inch from the top of the pans and bake 1½ hours or until interior temperature registers 190°F. on a meat thermometer. or Spread half of the turkey mixture in each of 2 greased steam table pans (12 × 20 × 2 inch) and bake 1¼ hours. 3. Let cooked loaf stand 5 to 10 minutes before slicing; serve with chicken gravy or mushroom sauce.

YIELD
50 portions

PORTION SIZE
4 ounces

PAN SIZE
Loaf pans or
12 × 20 × 2-inch steam table pans

TEMPERATURE
350°F. Oven

NOTE
1. If ground raw turkey is not available, grind raw turkey rolls or cubed raw turkey or bone out a large turkey and grind the meat, using a medium blade on the grinder.
2. The loaf mixture may also be shaped into 4 equal loaves and baked on a sheet pan, allowing about 1½ to 2 hours to bake, depending upon the thickness of the loaf.

DIETARY INFORMATION
May be used as written for general, bland, no added salt and mechanical soft diets. Diabetic diets — each serving provides 3 lean meat and 1/2 bread exchanges. Each serving provides 3 ounces cooked turkey and eggs.

YIELD
50 portions (2 pans)

PORTION SIZE
1 cup (8 ounces)

PAN SIZE
Heavy 3-gallon pot
12 × 20 x 2-inch steam table pans

DIETARY INFORMATION
May be used as written for general, bland, restricted residue, soft, and no added salt diets. Diabetic diets — each serving provides 4 lean meat and 1½ bread exchanges. Low cholesterol diets — omit eggs. Use 2 cups liquid egg substitute in step 5. Omit shortening and use ½ cup melted margarine or oil in step 6. Each serving provides 3 ounces cooked chicken or turkey.

Chicken or Turkey Pie with Batter Topping

Refer to footnotes for special dietary information

INGREDIENTS	WEIGHTS/MEASURES	YIELD ADJUST.	METHOD
Boiling water. . . . . 1½ gallons Chicken soup and gravy base. .as necessary			1. Prepare 1½ gallons chicken stock according to directions on the chicken soup and gravy base container.
Margarine, melted. . . . . .1½ cups (12 ounces) All-purpose flour . . . . .3 cups Celery salt . . . . .1 teaspoon			2. Combine margarine, flour and celery salt; mix until smooth; add to hot stock; cook and stir over medium heat until smooth and thickened and the starchy taste is gone.
Precooked diced chicken or turkey with skin and gristle removed . . . . .9 pounds, 8 ounces			3. Put half of the diced chicken or turkey in bottom of each of 2 steam table pans.
Drained canned peas and carrots. . . . . .3 quarts (1 No. 10 can) Diced cooked potatoes. . . . . . .1 quart			4. Stir peas and carrots and potatoes into hot sauce; then pour half of the mixture over chicken or turkey in each pan; mix lightly.
BATTER TOPPING: Slightly beaten eggs . . . . .2 cups (10 to 12 medium) Sugar. . . . . .1 tablespoon Milk . . . . .1 quart			5. Add eggs and sugar to milk and mix thoroughly.
All-purpose flour . . . . .3½ cups Baking powder . . . . .2 tablespoons Salt . . . . .1 tablespoon Shortening, melted . . . . .½ cup			6. Stir flour, baking powder and salt together; add egg mixture; mix lightly; add melted shortening; mix well. 7. Pour half of the batter over the top of chicken or turkey mixture in each pan. 8. Bake 20 to 30 minutes or until crust is golden brown.

Chicken or Turkey a la King

Refer to footnotes for special dietary information

INGREDIENTS	WEIGHTS/MEASURES	YIELD ADJUST.	METHOD
Canned drained mushrooms . . 1 16-ounce can			1. Fry mushrooms in margarine in a heavy pot, stirring constantly, for 1 or 2 minutes.
Margarine . . . . 1 cup (8 ounces)			2. Stir flour and salt into mushrooms; cook and stir until well blended but not brown.
All-purpose flour . . . . 2 cups			3. Stir cold milk into flour mixture; cook and stir over moderate heat about 10 to 15 minutes or until smooth and thickened and the starchy taste has disappeared.
Salt . . . . 2 tablespoons			
Cold milk. . . . . 1 gallon			
Sherry (optional) . . . . 1 cup			4. Add sherry, chicken or turkey and pimientos to the hot sauce; reheat over low heat; serve hot.
Precooked diced chicken or turkey with gristle and skin removed . . . . 9 pounds, 8 ounces			
Drained chopped pimientos . . . 1 cup			

YIELD
50 portions (about 2¼ gallons)

PORTION SIZE
¾ cup (6-ounce ladle)

PAN SIZE
Heavy 3-gallon pot

DIETARY INFORMATION
May be used as written by general, bland, residue restricted, soft and no added salt diets. Diabetic diets — each serving provides 3 lean meat and 1 skim milk exchanges. Each serving provides 3 ounces cooked chicken or turkey.

YIELD
50 portions (about 3¼ gallons)

PORTION SIZE
1 cup (8 ounces)

PAN SIZE
Heavy 5-gallon pot

NOTES
1. 6 pounds, 4 ounces chicken or turkey may be used instead of the 9 pounds, 8 ounces of chicken or turkey in step 3. If the 6 pounds, 4 ounces of chicken or turkey are used, each portion will provide 2 ounces of cooked chicken or turkey.
2. 4 pounds of macaroni may be used instead of the 4 pounds of egg noodles in step 1, if desired.

DIETARY INFORMATION
May be used as written for general and no added salt diets. Diabetic diets — each serving provides 4 lean meat and 2 bread exchanges. Bland and restricted residue diets — omit pepper. Low cholesterol diets — use margarine in step 2. Each serving provides 3 ounces cooked chicken or turkey.

Chicken or Turkey and Noodles

Refer to footnotes for special dietary information

INGREDIENTS	WEIGHTS/MEASURES	YIELD ADJUST.	METHOD
Boiling chicken stock	4 gallons		1. Stir noodles into boiling stock; return to a boil; cook 15 minutes or until noodles are tender. (Time will depend upon the size of the noodles.) If chicken stock is not available, prepare with hot water and chicken soup and gravy base.) Drain noodles; save 1½ gallons of hot stock for step 2. Do not wash the noodles.
Egg noodles, broken into short pieces	4 pounds		
Chicken fat or margarine, melted	¾ cup		2. Mix fat and flour together. Bring the 1½ gallons of the hot stock in which you cooked the noodles to a boil; stir flour mixture into hot stock; cook and stir until smooth and thickened and until the starchy taste is gone; add pepper and as much salt as necessary.
All-purpose flour	1½ cups		
White pepper	1 teaspoon		
Salt	as necessary		
Precooked diced chicken or turkey with skin and gristle removed	9 pounds 8 ounces		3. Stir noodles and chicken or turkey into hot sauce; mix well and reheat over low heat. Serve hot.

Chicken in Tomato Sauce

Refer to footnotes for special dietary information

INGREDIENTS	WEIGHTS/MEASURES	YIELD ADJUST.	METHOD
2 to 2½ pound broiler-fryers cut into 8 pieces . . . . .28 pounds			1. Wash chicken thoroughly under running cool water. Drain well. Pat chicken dry with a clean cloth or paper towels. Place chicken pieces, skin side up, on lightly greased sheet pans. Bake at 400°F. for about 1 hour or until browned. Place hot chicken in roaster. Discard fat and liquid in sheet pans.
Tomato sauce . . . . .4½ quarts (1½ No. 10 cans) Fat-free chicken broth. . . . . . .1½ quarts Italian seasoning . . . . .2 tablespoons Finely chopped onions. . . . . . .1 quart Salt . . . . .1 tablespoon			2. Place tomato sauce, broth, seasoning, onions and salt in pot. Bring to a boil, reduce heat and simmer, uncovered, for 20 minutes. Pour the hot sauce over the hot chicken in roaster. Stir lightly to distribute the sauce. Cover and bake at 325°F. for 1 hour. Remove the cover and continue to bake for another ½ hour or until the chicken is tender. Serve the chicken hot with some of the sauce over noodles or rice.

YIELD
50 portions

PORTION SIZE
2 pieces

PAN SIZE
18 × 26-inch sheet pans
Heavy 3-gallon pot
Roaster

TEMPERATURE
400°F. and 325°F. Oven

DIETARY INFORMATION
May be used as written for general, bland and no added salt diets. Diabetic diets — each serving provides 4 lean meat and ½ bread exchanges. Each serving provides 3 ounces cooked chicken.

YIELD
50 portions (about 3¼ gallons)

PORTION SIZE
1 cup (8 ounces)

PAN SIZE
Heavy 5-gallon pot
Roasting pan

TEMPERATURE
350°F. Oven

DIETARY INFORMATION
May be used as written for general and no added salt diets. Diabetic diets — each serving provides 4 lean meat and 2 bread exchanges. Bland diets — omit fresh green peppers and pepper. Each serving provides 3 ounces cooked turkey and cheese.

Chicken or Turkey Tetrazzini

Refer to footnotes for special dietary information

INGREDIENTS	WEIGHTS/MEASURES	YIELD ADJUST.	METHOD
Spaghetti	3 pounds		1. Stir spaghetti into boiling water; add vegetable oil; cook about 15 minutes or until tender; drain well but do not rinse with cold water. (Try to cook spaghetti so that it will still be warm when it is combined with the sauce.)
Boiling water	3 gallons		
Salt	3 tablespoons		
Vegetable oil	2 tablespoons		
Canned mushrooms	2 16-oz. cans		2. Drain mushrooms; save juice for use in step 4; chop mushrooms.
Chopped onions	¾ cup		3. Fry onions, fresh green peppers and mushrooms in butter or margarine until onions are golden.
Chopped fresh green peppers	¾ cup		
Margarine	¼ cup (2 ounces)		
Boiling hot chicken stock	1 gallon		4. Combine chicken stock and mushroom juice; stir dry milk into hot stock; stir to mix well.
Mushroom juice and water	2 quarts		
Instant dry milk	3 cups		
All-purpose flour	2 cups		5. Stir flour into melted fat; add to hot stock; cook and stir over moderate heat until smooth and thickened; add pepper and salt, if necessary; cook, stirring frequently, until starchy taste is gone.
Chicken fat or margarine, melted	1 cup		
White pepper	1 teaspoon		
Salt	as necessary		
Cubed Swiss cheese	2 pounds		6. Stir onion mixture, Swiss cheese and chicken or turkey into lukewarm sauce; add spaghetti, mix lightly; pour into well-greased roasting pan; sprinkle with Parmesan cheese; bake 30 to 40 minutes or until hot and bubbly and lightly browned.
Precooked diced chicken or turkey with skin and gristle removed	7 pounds, 6 ounces		
Grated Parmesan cheese	½ cup		

Chapter 6
Fish

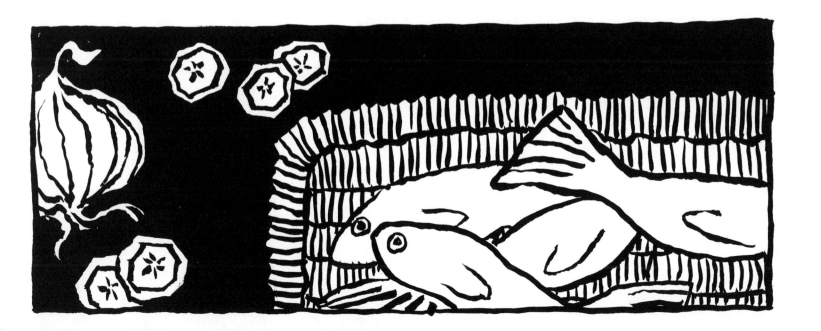

Fish Information

STORING AND THAWING FISH AND SHELLFISH

Storing

1. Canned fish and shellfish should be stored in a cool dry storage area.
2. Fresh fish and shellfish should be delivered packed in crushed ice. Fresh fish and shellfish should be stored in the refrigerator at 35° to 40°F. until removed for cooking
3. Do not hold fresh fish or shellfish longer than 1 day before it is cooked.
4. Frozen fish and shellfish should be delivered hard-frozen. Frozen fish and shellfish should be stored in the freezer at 0°F. or colder until it is removed for thawing. Frozen fish or shellfish should be used within 1 month.

Thawing

1. Thawing should be scheduled so that fish or shellfish will be cooked soon after it is thawed. Do not hold thawed fish or shellfish longer than 1 day before cooking it.
2. Remove only the amount of fish or shellfish needed for 1 day's use from the freezer at a time.
3. Remove fish from the cartons and place individual packages or cans on trays in the refrigerator at 35° to 40°F. to thaw. Allow 24 to 36 hours for thawing 1-pound packages or cans and 48 to 72 hours for thawing the 5-pound or gallon cans.
4. If quicker thawing is necessary, remove the fish from the cartons and thaw the individual packages in cold water. Change the water often to speed the thawing. Use cold water. DO NOT USE HOT WATER FOR THAWING FISH OR SHELLFISH. Allow 1 to 2 hours for thawing 1-pound packages and 2 to 3 hours for thawing 5-pound packages. Allow 6 to 8 hours for thawing gallon cans.
5. DO NOT THAW FISH AT ROOM TEMPERATURE.
6. DO NOT REFREEZE FISH WHICH HAS BEEN THAWED.
7. FISH PORTIONS AND FISH STICKS SHOULD NOT BE THAWED BEFORE THEY ARE COOKED. Remove only the amounts needed for that meal from the freezer.
8. Frozen fillets and steaks may be cooked without thawing but it will take longer to cook them. Fillets or steaks to be breaded or stuffed should always be thawed.

Fish should be cooked as close to serving time as possible and should not be transferred from one pan to another any more than absolutely necessary because it is very tender and breaks easily.

Fish and shellfish must be properly handled during storage, thawing, preparation, cooking and serving in order to avoid spoilage or food poisoning.

LEFTOVER COOKED FISH

1. Leftover cooked fish should be stored in the refrigerator or freezer. If stored in the refrigerator, it should be stored in a covered pan and used within 4 days. If stored in the freezer, it should be sealed in a moisture-proof bag, wrapped in freezer paper or aluminum foil and used within 1 month.
2. Leftover cooked fish may be flaked and used in fish salads, combined with barbecue sauce for an attractive hot sandwich or mixed with a medium white sauce for creamed fish.

Baked Fish Creole

Refer to footnotes for special dietary information

YIELD
50 portions (2 pans)

PORTION SIZE
1 piece plus sauce

PAN SIZE
12 x 20 x 2-inch steam table pans

TEMPERATURE
350°F. Oven

DIETARY INFORMATION
May be used as written for general, low cholesterol and no added salt diets. Diabetic diets — each serving provides 3 lean meat and 1 vegetable exchanges. Bland diets — omit fresh green peppers, pepper and cloves. Each serving provides 3 ounces cooked fish.

INGREDIENTS	WEIGHTS/MEASURES	YIELD ADJUST.	METHOD
Fish fillets or steaks (perch, cod, flounder, haddock, pollock, rockfish or whiting)	.12 pounds, 8 ounces (50 4-oz. each)		1. Thaw fish, if necessary; place in a single layer (skin side down, if applicable) in greased steam table pans.
Finely chopped onions	.2 cups		2. Fry onions and green peppers in margarine until onions are golden.
Chopped fresh green peppers	.2 cups		
Margarine	.¾ cup (6 ounces)		
All-purpose flour	.1 cup		3. Stir flour into onion mixture; cook and stir over low heat until smooth.
Canned crushed tomatoes	.3 quarts (1 No. 10 can)		4. Add tomatoes, salt, pepper, sugar and cloves to flour mixture; cook, stirring occasionally, until thickened.
Salt	.2 tablespoons		5. Pour half of the hot sauce over fish in each pan.
Pepper	.½ teaspoon		
Sugar	.2 tablespoons		6. Bake 30 to 40 minutes or until fish flakes easily.
Ground cloves	.¼ teaspoon		

YIELD
50 portions

PORTION SIZE
1 steak

PAN SIZE
Baking pans

TEMPERATURE
350°F. Oven

VARIATION
Italian-style baked halibut or salmon:
Use about 3 cups Italian-style vinegar
and oil dressing to brush fish in step 2
instead of oil, lemon juice, onions, salt
and pepper.

DIETARY INFORMATION
May be used as written for general, low
cholesterol and no added salt diets.
Diabetic diets — each serving provides
3 lean meat exchanges. Bland diets —
omit pepper. Each serving provides 3
ounces cooked fish.

Baked Halibut or Salmon Steak

Refer to footnotes for special dietary information

INGREDIENTS	WEIGHTS/MEASURES	YIELD ADJUST.	METHOD
Halibut or salmon steaks	12 pounds, 8 ounces (50 4-oz. steaks)		1. Thaw frozen fish, if necessary; divide into 4-ounce steaks; place in a single layer in well-greased baking pans.
Vegetable oil . . . . .1 cup Lemon juice . . . . .¾ cup Finely chopped onions . . . . . . .1 cup Salt . . . . .2 tablespoons Pepper. . . . . .½ teaspoon Lemon slices. 50			2. Combine oil, lemon juice, onions, salt and pepper; mix well; brush fish generously with oil mixture using a pastry brush. 3. Bake 25 to 35 minutes or until fish flakes easily when tested with a fork; serve hot with lemon slice.

Baked Fish with Egg Sauce

Refer to footnotes for special dietary information

INGREDIENTS	WEIGHTS/MEASURES	YIELD ADJUST.	METHOD
Fish fillets or steaks (perch, cod, flounder, haddock, pollock, rockfish or whiting) .12 pounds, 8 ounces (50 4-oz. each)			1. Thaw fish, if necessary, and place in a single layer (skin-side down, if applicable) in greased pans.
Vegetable oil . . . . .1 cup Lemon juice . . . . .1 cup Salt .3 tablespoons Pepper. . . . . .1 teaspoon Paprika . . . . .2 tablespoons			2. Combine oil, lemon juice, salt, pepper and paprika. Brush fish generously with oil mixture using a pastry brush. 3. Bake 25 to 35 minutes or until fish flakes easily when tested with a fork. 4. Serve hot with ¼ cup (2-ounce ladle) of hot egg sauce.
EGG SAUCE: Margarine, melted. . . . . .½ cup (1 stick) All-purpose flour . . . . .1 cup Salt .1 tablespoon Dry mustard . . . . .1 tablespoon Cold milk. . . . . .2 quarts			5. Stir flour, salt and mustard into melted fat; cook and stir until smooth but not browned. 6. Add cold milk to flour mixture; cook and stir until smooth and thickened and the starchy taste is gone.
Chopped hard-cooked eggs . . .12 Chopped parsley. . . . . .½ cup			7. Add eggs and parsley to sauce; serve ¼ cup (2-ounce ladle) hot sauce over each portion of fish.

YIELD
50 portions (2 pans)

PORTION SIZE
1 piece plus
2-ounce ladle of sauce

PAN SIZE
12 × 20 × 2-inch steam table pans
Heavy saucepan

TEMPERATURE
350°F. Oven

DIETARY INFORMATION
May be used as written for general and no added salt diets. Diabetic diets — each serving provides 3 ½ lean meat and 1 vegetable exchanges. Bland diets — omit pepper. Each serving provides 3 ounces cooked fish.

YIELD
50 portions

PORTION SIZE
1 fillet

PAN SIZE
18 × 26-inch sheet pans

TEMPERATURE
475°F. Oven

DIETARY INFORMATION
May be used as written for general, bland and no added salt diets. Diabetic diets — each serving provides 3 lean meat and 1 vegetable exchanges. Each serving provides 3 ounces cooked fish.

Oven-Fried Fish Fillets

Refer to footnotes for special dietary information

INGREDIENTS	WEIGHTS/MEASURES	YIELD ADJUST.	METHOD
Fish fillets (perch, cod, flounder, haddock, pollock, rockfish or whiting)	12 pounds, 8 ounces (50 4-oz. fillets)		1. Thaw frozen fillets, if necessary.
Salt . . . . Milk . . . . Dry bread crumbs . . . . Garlic powder	1 tablespoon 2 cups 1 quart (1 pound) ½ teaspoon		2. Add salt to milk. 3. Combine crumbs and garlic powder; mix well. 4. Dip fillets first in milk and then in crumbs; put in a single layer on well-greased sheet pans.
Vegetable oil	1 cup		5. Sprinkle or pour oil over fish, being sure to get a little bit of oil on each piece of fish. 6. Bake 20 to 25 minutes or until fish is browned and flakes easily when tested with a fork.

Tuna Macaroni Loaf

Refer to footnotes for special dietary information

INGREDIENTS	WEIGHTS/MEASURES	YIELD ADJUST.	METHOD
Macaroni	3 pounds, 8 ounces (3½ quarts)		1. Stir macaroni into boiling salted water; return to a boil; add oil; cook, uncovered, about 6 minutes or until not quite tender. Drain well but do not rinse.
Boiling water	3½ gallons		
Salt	3 tablespoons		
Vegetable oil	2 tablespoons		
Canned tunafish	4-pound can		2. Drain tunafish well; discard oil or water; break up tunafish with a fork.
Soft bread crumbs	2 pounds (3 quarts)		3. Add tunafish, bread crumbs and olives to hot macaroni; mix lightly.
Sliced pimiento-stuffed green olives	1 quart		
Condensed cheese soup	3 quarts (2 46-oz. cans)		4. Combine soup, milk, eggs, garlic salt and mustard; pour over macaroni mixture; stir gently to mix well; pour half of the mixture into each of 2 greased steam table pans.
Milk	1 gallon		5. Bake 45 to 60 minutes or until firm.
Beaten eggs	3 cups (15 to 18 medium)		6. Cut each pan 4 × 6.
Garlic salt	3 tablespoons		
Dry mustard	2 tablespoons		

YIELD
48 portions (2 pans)

PORTION SIZE
7 ounces

PAN SIZE
Heavy 5-gallon pot
12 × 20 × 2-inch steam table pans

TEMPERATURE
350°F. Oven

DIETARY INFORMATION
May be used as written for general, bland and mechanical soft diets. Diabetic diets — each serving provides 2 medium fat meat and 1½ bread exchanges. No added salt diets — omit olives in step 3. Add 1 cup cooked pimientos instead of the olives. Each serving provides 2 ounces cooked tunafish, eggs and cheese.

YIELD
50 portions (2 pans)

PORTION SIZE
¾ cup (6 ounces)

PAN SIZE
12 × 20 × 2-inch steam table pans

TEMPERATURE
350°F. Oven

NOTE
3 pounds of macaroni may be used instead of the noodles in step 1, if desired. Cook macaroni according to directions on the package, until barely tender.

DIETARY INFORMATION
May be used as written for general, bland, no added salt and mechanical soft diets. Diabetic diets — each serving provides 1 bread, 1 vegetable, 1 lowfat milk, and 2 lean meat exchanges. Each serving provides 2 ounces cooked tunafish.

Tunafish, Noodles and Mushrooms

Refer to footnotes for special dietary information

INGREDIENTS	WEIGHTS/MEASURES	YIELD ADJUST.	METHOD
Noodles.................3 pounds Boiling water.............5 gallons Salt ....3 tablespoons			1. Drop noodles into boiling, salted water; stir lightly to mix. Add oil and cook, uncovered, over medium heat, about 12 minutes or until noodles are tender. Drain noodles well; rinse with cold water and save for use in step 4.

Condensed cream of
   mushroom soup ....3 quarts
   (2 46-ounce cans)
Milk ....2 quarts
			2. Combine soup and milk and mix together until smooth.

Canned tunafish...........7 pounds
   (1¾ 4-pound
   cans)
Canned mushrooms........2 1-pound
   cans
			3. Drain tunafish and mushrooms well. Discard oil and/or liquid. Break up the tunafish with a fork.
			4. Add tunafish and mushrooms to soup mixture; stir lightly to mix well; add to drained noodles and stir lightly to mix.
			5. Place half of the noodle mixture into each of 2 buttered steam table pans.

Dry bread crumbs ....1 quart
   (1 pound)
Margarine, melted..........1 cup
   (8 ounces)
Grated Parmesan cheese .....1 cup
Paprika ....1 tablespoon
			6. Combine crumbs, margarine, Parmesan cheese and paprika; mix well. Sprinkle half of the crumb mixture over each of the 2 pans of the noodle mixture.
			7. Bake 30 to 45 minutes or until lightly browned and bubbly. Serve hot.

Creamed Tunafish

Refer to footnotes for special dietary information

INGREDIENTS	WEIGHTS/MEASURES	YIELD ADJUST.	METHOD
Canned tunafish . . . . .6 pounds (1½ 4-pound cans)			1. Drain and flake tunafish. If the fish is canned in oil, reserve oil and use it for part of the fat in step 2.
Margarine, melted, or oil from the tunafish. . . . . .1¼ cups All-purpose flour . . . . .2½ cups			2. Blend fat and flour together and stir until smooth.
Nonfat dry milk . . . . .1¾ quarts Hot water . . . . .1¼ gallons			3. Stir milk into hot water; heat to just below boiling. DO NOT BOIL. 4. Add flour mixture to hot milk, stirring constantly; add salt and simmer 10 to 15 minutes over low heat until thickened and smooth, stirring occasionally.
Chopped pimiento . . . . .1 cup Worcestershire sauce. . . . . . . .¼ cup Garlic salt . . . . .1 teaspoon White pepper. . . . . .½ teaspoon Salt . . . . .2 tablespoons Chopped hard-cooked eggs . . .12			5. Add pimientos, Worcestershire sauce, garlic salt, pepper, salt, eggs and flaked tunafish to white sauce; reheat over low heat; serve hot.

YIELD
50 portions (about 2¼ gallons)

PORTION SIZE
¾ cup (6-ounce ladle)

PAN SIZE
Heavy 3-gallon pot

DIETARY INFORMATION
May be used as written for general, no added salt and mechanical soft diets. Diabetic diets — each serving provides 1 milk and 2 lean meat exchanges. Bland diets — omit pepper. Each serving provides 2 ounces cooked tunafish.

Salmon Patties with Creamed Peas

Refer to footnotes for special dietary information

YIELD
50 portions

PORTION SIZE
1 salmon patty
1/2 cup creamed peas

PAN SIZE
18 × 26-inch sheet pans
Heavy 3-gallon pot

TEMPERATURE
400° F. Oven

DIETARY INFORMATION
May be used as written for general, no added salt, mechanical soft and bland diets. Diabetic diets — each salmon patty without sauce provides 2 medium fat meat and 1/2 bread exchanges. Each salmon patty with 1/2 cup creamed peas provides 2 medium fat meat, 1 vegetable and 1/2 bread exchanges. Each serving provides 2 ounces cooked salmon.

INGREDIENTS	WEIGHTS/MEASURES	YIELD ADJUST.	METHOD
Canned salmon	8 1-pound cans		1. Drain salmon well. Discard skin and bones and place salmon and juice in mixer bowl.
Crushed soda crackers	2 quarts (1 pound)		2. Add crackers, eggs, onions and milk to salmon. Mix at low speed to blend. Do not beat. Let stand 5 minutes.
Slightly beaten eggs	2 cups (10 to 12 medium)		
Minced instant dry onions	1 cup		
Milk	2 3/4 cups		
Softened margarine	1/2 cup (4 ounces)		3. Spread margarine evenly over the bottom of the sheet pan. 4. Using a No. 12 dipper, place mounds of salmon mixture on the sheet pan, leaving room to flatten the mound. 5. Bake 15 to 20 minutes or until golden brown on the bottom. Turn mounds over and flatten each one to form a salmon patty about 3 1/2 inches wide. Bake 10 minutes longer. Serve hot with creamed peas.
CREAMED PEAS: Canned peas	3 quarts (1 No. 10 can)		1. Drain peas, reserving 2 cups of the liquid. Combine peas, liquid and margarine and heat to simmering. 2. Combine flour and milk and stir until smooth. Add to peas and cook and stir over moderate heat until smooth and thickened. Serve hot over salmon patties.
Margarine	1 cup (8 ounces)		
All-purpose flour	1 1/2 cups		
Milk	2 1/2 quarts		

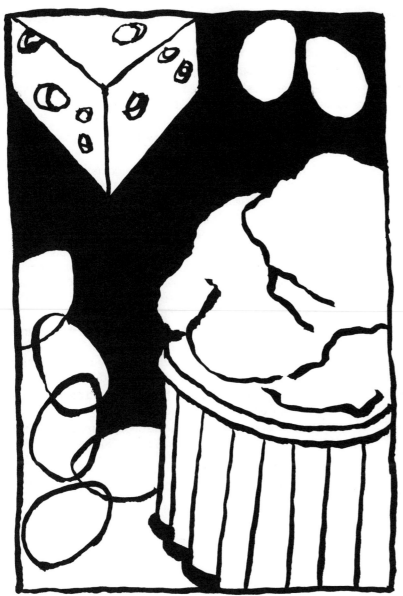

Chapter 7
Cheese and Eggs

Cheese and Egg Information

PROPER USE OF CHEESE

1. Low to moderate temperatures should always be used for cooking cheese. High heat or extended cooking time will cause cheese to become dry, rubbery, stringy and tough or it may cause the cheese to separate which will cause the finished food to be oily.

2. It is a good idea to use a double boiler in the preparation of cheese sauce.

3. Cheese is cooked when it is melted. A cheese sauce does not need to cook any longer after the cheese is melted and it may become stringy or the cheese may separate if it is cooked longer.

4. Cheese should be kept refrigerated in a tightly covered container or wrapped in wax paper, plastic wrap or aluminum foil and refrigerated. Small chunks of leftover cheese can be combined and ground together to be used as a topping for casseroles or added to a cheese sauce.

5. Mold may form on any natural bulk cheese. The mold is not harmful but should be cut off before the cheese is served.

6. Cheese is high in protein. One-fourth cup cottage cheese or 1 ounce other cheeses will provide an ounce of protein in the daily diet.

PROPER USE OF EGGS

1. Eggs should always be kept refrigerated or in a very cool place. They should never be frozen in their shells although shelled frozen eggs may be used instead of whole fresh eggs. Frozen eggs have the same nutritive value as fresh eggs and are very handy to use.

2. Grade A medium eggs are generally purchased for most uses.

3. Eggs are easily digested by most people and are generally well-accepted as a part of their daily diet. Eggs are a valuable source of protein and 1 egg provides an ounce of protein in the daily diet.

4. Eggs should be cooked with low heat. Cooking eggs with high heat will toughen the egg white.

5. Eggs should be removed from the refrigerator about 1/2 hour before they are used. This will help prevent cracked shells when they are hard-cooked and will result in a better volume when used for beaten egg whites.

6. Each egg should be broken separately into a small dish before it is added to other ingredients. If an egg has a bad odor, appearance or color, it can then be discarded without spoiling the rest of the ingredients.

7. Hard-cooked eggs should be covered with cold running water as soon as they finish cooking to prevent the yolks from discoloring and to make the shells easier to remove. They should be thoroughly chilled before they are drained and put into the refrigerator.

8. Hard-cooked eggs should not be shelled until they are to be used to prevent darkening and to avoid bacterial contamination. When they have been shelled, they should be put into a colander or sieve and dipped into boiling water for 30 seconds to 1 minute to destroy any bacteria.

9. Egg yolks will not crumble when slicing hard-cooked eggs, if you dip the knife in cold water before they are sliced.

10. Hard-cooked eggs should not be chopped for salad until time to put them into the salad to prevent bacterial contamination.

Baked Cheese Sandwich

Refer to footnotes for special dietary information

INGREDIENTS	WEIGHTS/MEASURES	YIELD ADJUST.	METHOD
Day-old white bread . . . . .90 slices Processed American cheese . .4 pounds, 4 ounces (68 1-ounce slices)			1. Arrange 15 slices of bread in the bottom of each well-greased steam table pan. 2. Put 1½ slices of cheese on each slice of bread; cover with remaining bread.
Skim milk . . . . .1¼ gallons Eggs .36 Dry mustard . . . . .1 tablespoon Salt . . . . .2 tablespoons Paprika . . . . .1 tablespoon			3. Combine milk, eggs, mustard, salt and paprika; beat with a wire whip or egg beater until smooth; pour ⅓ of the mixture over sandwiches in each pan; refrigerate 1 hour. 4. Bake 45 minutes to 1 hour or until puffed and golden brown.

YIELD
45 portions (3 pans)

PORTION SIZE
1 sandwich

PAN SIZE
12 × 20 × 2-inch steam table pans

TEMPERATURE
325°F. Oven

DIETARY INFORMATION
May be used as written for general, bland, soft and no added salt diets. Diabetic diets — each serving provides 2 bread and 2 high fat meat exchanges. Each serving provides 2 ounces of cheese and eggs.

YIELD
48 portions (2 pans)

PORTION SIZE
1 square

PAN SIZE
12 × 20 × 2-inch steam table pans

TEMPERATURE
325°F. Oven

DIETARY INFORMATION
May be used as written for general, bland, soft and no added salt diets. Diabetic diets — each serving provides 1½ bread and 2 high fat meat exchanges. Each serving provides 2 ounces of cheese and eggs.

Cheese Fondue

Refer to footnotes for special dietary information

INGREDIENTS	WEIGHTS/MEASURES	YIELD ADJUST.	METHOD
Nonfat dry milk . . . . .3 cups Hot water . . . . .2½ quarts			1. Stir dry milk into hot water; cool to lukewarm.
Eggs .1 quart (20-24 medium) Salt .1 tablespoon Grated American process or cheddar cheese . . . . .5 pounds			2. Beat eggs thoroughly in mixer bowl; add milk; mix well. 3. Add salt and cheese to egg mixture; mix lightly.
Fresh bread cubes . . . . .3 pounds (about 1 gallon)			4. Add bread cubes to cheese and milk mixture; pour ½ of the mixture into each of 2 well-buttered pans; refrigerate until baked. (This may be prepared 2 or 3 hours before baking, if desired.) 5. Bake about 45 minutes or until firm and lightly browned. 6. Cut each pan 4 × 6.

Cheese, Rice and Olive Squares with Cheese Sauce

Refer to footnotes for special dietary information

INGREDIENTS	WEIGHTS/MEASURES	YIELD ADJUST.	METHOD
Long grain rice	2 pounds, 12 ounces (1½ quarts)		1. Combine rice, cold water, salt and oil in a heavy pot; bring to a boil, stirring occasionally; cover tightly; simmer 15 minutes. DO NOT STIR. If rice is not tender, cover and cook 2 to 3 minutes longer.
Cold water................	3 quarts		
Salt	3 tablespoons		
Vegetable oil	2 tablespoons		2. Uncover rice and allow it to stand for at least 10 minutes.
Nonfat dry milk............	1½ cups		3. Stir dry milk into water; heat to just below boiling point but do not boil.
Warm water...............	1¼ quarts		
All-purpose flour...........	¾ cup		4. Stir flour and salt into melted margarine; mix until smooth; add to hot milk, stirring constantly using a wire whip, cook until smooth and thickened.
Salt	1 teaspoon		
Margarine, melted..........	¾ cup (6 ounces)		
Ground or shredded cheddar or American process cheese ..	1 pound, 8 ounces		5. Add cheese to hot sauce; stir until smooth; add to rice; mix well; cool slightly.
Egg yolks	30		6. Beat egg yolks until creamy and light yellow; add mustard, salt and paprika; add egg yolks and olives to cheese and rice mixture; mix well.
Dry mustard	2 tablespoons		
Salt	1 tablespoon		
Paprika	1 tablespoon		
Sliced pimiento-stuffed green olives..................	3 cups		
Egg whites	30		7. Beat egg whites until they form soft peaks; fold carefully into rice mixture.
			8. Pour ½ of the mixture into each of 2 well-greased steam table pans; bake 45 minutes or until firm and lightly browned; cut each pan 4 by 6.

YIELD
48 portions (2 pans)

PORTION SIZE
1 square plus
½ cup cheese sauce

PAN SIZE
Heavy 3-gallon pot
12 × 20 × 2-inch steam table pans

TEMPERATURE
325°F. Oven

NOTE
Tomato sauce or mushroom sauce may be served with squares instead of cheese sauce, if desired.

DIETARY INFORMATION
May be used as written for general, bland and no added salt diets. Diabetic diets — each serving provides 2 bread, 2 high fat meat and 1 fat exchanges. Each serving provides 2 ounces cheese and eggs.

Continues on next page

Continued from preceding page

INGREDIENTS	WEIGHTS/MEASURES	YIELD ADJUST.	METHOD
CHEESE SAUCE: All-purpose flour . . . . .2 cups Salt . . . . .2 tablespoons Margarine, melted. . . . . .1 cup (8 ounces)			9. Stir flour and salt into melted margarine; stir until smooth.
Nonfat dry milk . . . . .1¼ quarts Warm water . . . . .1¼ gallons			10. Stir dry milk into warm water; heat to just below boiling but do not boil; stir flour mixture into hot milk; cook and stir over moderate heat until smooth and thickened; continue to cook, stirring occasionally, using a wire whip, over low heat about 10 minutes or until the starchy taste is gone.
Ground or shredded cheddar or American process cheese . .3 pounds Worcestershire sauce . . . . . . .2 tablespoons			11. Add cheese and Worcestershire sauce to hot sauce; stir until smooth; serve hot over hot omelet.

Macaroni and Cheese

Refer to footnotes for special dietary information

INGREDIENTS	WEIGHTS/MEASURES	YIELD ADJUST.	METHOD
Elbow macaroni . . . . .3 pounds (3 quarts) Boiling water. . . . . .3 gallons Salt .3 tablespoons Vegetable oil . . . . .2 tablespoons			1. Stir macaroni into boiling salted water; add oil; cook 10 to 12 minutes or until tender, stirring occasionally; drain well.
Nonfat dry milk. . . . . .1¼ quarts Warm water. . . . . .1¼ gallons			2. Stir milk into water; heat to just below boiling point but do not boil.
All-purpose flour . . . . .1½ cups Salt .2 tablespoons Pepper. . . . . .1 teaspoon Dry mustard . . . . .1 tablespoon Margarine, melted. . . . . .1 cup (8 ounces)			3. Stir flour, salt, pepper and mustard into melted margarine; mix until smooth; add to hot milk, stirring constantly with a wire whip; cook until smooth and thickened.
Ground or shredded cheddar or American process cheese . .4 pounds			4. Add cheese to sauce; stir until smooth; add to macaroni; mix well. 5. Put half of the macaroni mixture into each of 2 well-greased pans.
Dry bread crumbs . . . . .3 cups Margarine, melted. . . . . .½ cup Paprika . . . . .as necessary			6. Combine crumbs and melted margarine; sprinkle ½ of the mixture over macaroni in each pan; sprinkle lightly with paprika. 7. Bake 30 to 45 minutes or until lightly browned.

YIELD
50 portions (2 pans)

PORTION SIZE
¾ cup (6 ounces)

PAN SIZE
Heavy 5-gallon pot
12 × 20 × 2-inch steam table pan

TEMPERATURE
350°F. Oven

VARIATIONS
1. Macaroni with cheese and ham: Add 3 pounds diced, canned ham to cheese sauce in step 4. Each portion of this recipe will provide 2 ounces protein.
2. Baked macaroni with cheese and pimiento: Add 1 cup diced pimiento to cheese sauce in step 4.
3. Baked macaroni and cheese with tomatoes: Add 1 quart peeled, diced, drained fresh tomatoes to macaroni and sauce in step 4.

DIETARY INFORMATION
May be used as written for general and no added salt diets. Diabetic diets — each serving provides 2 bread and 2 high fat meat exchanges. Bland diets — omit pepper. Each serving provides 1 ounce of cheese.

YIELD
50 portions (2 steam table pans)

PORTION SIZE
1 cup (8 ounces)

PAN SIZE
Heavy 5-gallon pot
12 × 20 × 2-inch steam table pan

TEMPERATURE
350°F. Oven

DIETARY INFORMATION
May be used as written for general, bland and no added salt diets. Diabetic diets — each serving provides 2 bread, 2 high fat meat and 1 fat exchanges. Each serving provides 2 ounces cheese.

Macaroni and Cheese with Olives

Refer to footnotes for special dietary information

INGREDIENTS	WEIGHTS/MEASURES	YIELD ADJUST.	METHOD
Elbow macaroni . . . . .4 pounds (1 gallon) Boiling water. . . . . .4 gallons Salt . . . . .¼ cup Vegetable oil . . . . .2 tablespoons			1. Stir macaroni into boiling salted water; add oil, cook 10 to 12 minutes or until tender; drain well.
Nonfat dry milk . . . . .3 cups All-purpose flour . . . . .1½ cups Salt . . . . .2 tablespoons Ground mustard . . . . .2 tablespoons Cold water. . . . . .1 quart			2. Combine dry milk, flour, salt and mustard; mix well; stir into cold water and mix to form a smooth paste.
Boiling water. . . . . .1 gallon			3. Stir flour mixture into boiling water; cook and stir over low heat until thickened and smooth; continue to cook and stir over low heat 2 or 3 minutes longer.
Ground or shredded American process cheese. . . . . .3 pounds Worcestershire sauce. . . . . . .2 tablespoons			4. Add cheese and Worcestershire sauce to thickened sauce; stir over low heat until cheese is melted; remove from heat; add macaroni to the cheese sauce and cool to lukewarm.
Cubed cheddar cheese. . . . . .3 pounds, 4 ounces Sliced pimiento-stuffed green olives. . . . . .1½ quarts Paprika . . . . .as necessary			5. Add cubed cheese and olives to cooled macaroni mixture; put half of the mixture into each of 2 buttered steam table pans. 6. Sprinkle each pan with paprika and bake, uncovered, 20 to 30 minutes or until heated through; serve hot.

Scalloped Noodles with Cheese, Tomatoes and Bacon

Refer to footnotes for special dietary information

INGREDIENTS	WEIGHTS/MEASURES	YIELD ADJUST.	METHOD
Chopped bacon . . . . .1 pound			1. Fry bacon until transparent but not quite crisp; drain well; discard fat.
Canned, crushed tomatoes . . .4½ quarts (1½ No. 10 cans) Salt .3 tablespoons Mixed Italian seasoning . . . . . .1 tablespoon			2. Combine tomatoes, salt and Italian seasoning; simmer, uncovered, 30 minutes.
Noodles. . . . . .4 pounds Boiling water. . . . . .2 gallons Salt .3 tablespoons Vegetable oil . . . . .2 tablespoons			3. Stir noodles into boiling salted water; mix well; add oil; cook 12 to 15 minutes or until tender; drain well. Add bacon and tomatoes to noodles; mix thoroughly.
Ground or shredded cheddar or American process cheese . .3 pounds Paprika . . . . .as necessary			4. Arrange alternate layers of noodle mixture and cheese in well-greased roasting pan; sprinkle with paprika; bake 25 to 30 minutes.

YIELD
50 portions (about 3¼ gallons)

PORTION SIZE
1 cup (8 ounces)

PAN SIZE
Heavy 5-gallon pot
Roasting pan

TEMPERATURE
350°F. Oven

DIETARY INFORMATION
May be used as written for general and bland diets. Diabetic diets — each serving provides 2 bread, 1 medium fat meat and 1 fat exchanges. Each serving provides 1 ounce cheese.

YIELD
50 portions

PORTION SIZE
1 egg (No. 16 dipper)

PAN SIZE
12 × 20 × 2-inch steam table pan

TEMPERATURE
350°F. Oven

VARIATION
Scrambled eggs with ham: Add 1 pound diced, canned ham to egg mixture before baking; stir lightly and bake as directed in step 3.

NOTE
This recipe yields 1 egg per person. If 2 eggs per person are scheduled, double the recipe and give each person 2 No. 16 or 1 No. 8 dipper of scrambled eggs.

DIETARY INFORMATION
May be used as written for general, bland, restricted residue, soft, no added salt and mechanical soft diets. Diabetic diets — each serving provides 1 medium fat meat exchange. Each serving provides 1 egg.

Baked Scrambled Eggs

Refer to footnotes for special dietary information

INGREDIENTS	WEIGHTS/MEASURES	YIELD ADJUST.	METHOD
Eggs ....50 medium Salt ....1½ tablespoons Skim milk ....3 cups			1. Beat eggs only until well blended; add salt and milk; mix well.
Margarine, melted..........½ cup (4 ounces)			2. Pour melted margarine into steam table pan; use a pastry brush to spread margarine on bottom and sides of the pan. 3. Pour beaten eggs into pan; bake about 20 minutes, stirring every 5 minutes.

Cooked Eggs

Refer to footnotes for special dietary information

INGREDIENTS	WEIGHTS/MEASURES	YIELD ADJUST.	METHOD
HARD-COOKED EGGS: Eggs . . . . .50 medium Hot water . . . . .as necessary			1. Cover eggs with hot water; simmer 10 to 15 minutes. DO NOT BOIL. 2. Remove eggs from water; serve immediately.
SOFT-COOKED EGGS: Eggs . . . . .50 medium Hot water . . . . .as necessary			1. Cover eggs with hot water; simmer 4 minutes. DO NOT BOIL. 2. Remove eggs from water; serve immediately.
STEAMER METHOD FOR COOKING EGGS: Eggs (broken) . . . . .50 medium			1. Put eggs in greased pan; be sure there are enough eggs in pan so whites cover yolks; do not cover pan; cook at 15 pounds pressure for 7 minutes. 2. Remove pan from steamer; cut eggs for easy removal. 3. Consistency of eggs can be controlled by adjusting time in steamer. 4. This is an excellent way to cook eggs for salads.

YIELD
50 portions

PORTION SIZE
1 egg

DIETARY INFORMATION
May be used as written for general, bland, no added salt, soft, restricted residue, low fat and mechanical soft diets. Diabetic diets — each egg provides 1 medium fat meat exchange. Each serving provides 1 egg.

YIELD
50 portions

PORTION SIZE
1 egg

PAN SIZE
12 × 20 × 2-inch steam table pan

DIETARY INFORMATION
May be used as written for general, bland, no added salt, soft, restricted residue, low fat and mechanical soft diets. Diabetic diets — each egg provides 1 medium fat meat exchange. Each serving provides 1 egg.

Poached Eggs

Refer to footnotes for special dietary information

INGREDIENTS	WEIGHTS/MEASURES	YIELD ADJUST.	METHOD
Eggs	50 medium		1. Break eggs, one at a time, into small dishes.
Water	3 quarts		2. Bring water to a boil in a greased steam table pan; reduce heat to a simmer and carefully add eggs.
			3. Cook eggs 3 to 5 minutes or until whites are set and yolks are covered with a white film.
			4. Lift eggs out of pan with a perforated skimmer; drain briefly by holding skimmer over pan while counting to 3 and serve immediately.

Creamed Eggs

Refer to footnotes for special dietary information

INGREDIENTS	WEIGHTS/MEASURES	YIELD ADJUST.	METHOD
Nonfat dry milk............3½ cups Warm water...............4½ quarts			1. Stir dry milk into water; heat to just below boiling. DO NOT BOIL.
Margarine, melted...........1 cup All-purpose flour............3 cups Salt.......................2 tablespoons			2. Mix melted margarine, flour and salt together; stir until smooth; add to milk, stirring constantly; cook and stir over low heat for 5 to 10 minutes or until thickened and the starchy taste is gone.
Hard-cooked eggs..........75			3. Cut eggs into fourths; add gently to sauce; reheat over low heat, stirring very gently only as much as necessary; serve hot.

YIELD
50 portions (about 2¼ gallons)

PORTION SIZE
¾ cup (6-ounce ladle)

PAN SIZE
Heavy 3-gallon pot

DIETARY INFORMATION
May be used as written for general, bland, restricted residue, no added salt, soft and mechanical soft diets. Diabetic diets — each serving provides ½ bread and 2 medium fat meat exchanges. Each serving provides 1½ ounces cheese and eggs.

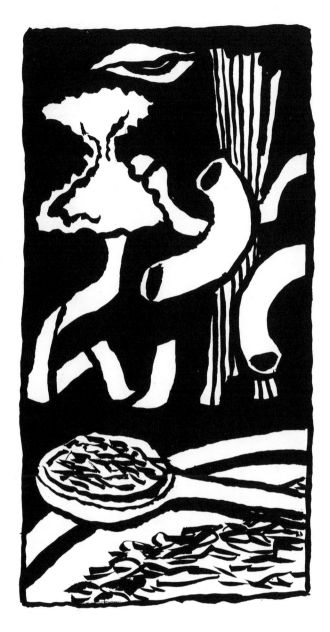

Chapter 8
Potatoes, Spaghetti and Rice

YIELD
50 portions (50 potatoes or yams)

PORTION SIZE
1 potato or yam

PAN SIZE
18 × 26-inch sheet pan

TEMPERATURE
400°F. Oven

DIETARY INFORMATION
May be used as written for general, no added salt, bland, low fat, low cholesterol, soft and mechanical soft diets. Diabetic diets — ¼ cup cooked or ½ small baked sweet potato or yam provides 1 bread exchange.

Baked Sweet Potatoes or Yams

Refer to footnotes for special dietary information

INGREDIENTS	WEIGHTS/MEASURES	YIELD ADJUST.	METHOD
Medium-size fresh sweet potatoes or yams	.50 (about 18 pounds, 12 ounces)		1. Scrub sweet potatoes or yams thoroughly. Cut off the ends and any bad spots; pierce in two or three places with a heavy fork or thin knife. Place on lightly greased sheet pan. Do not crowd them. 2. Bake about 1 hour or until they feel soft when they are squeezed. Slit the top of the yam or sweet potato crosswise and open slightly. Serve hot.

Candied Sweet Potatoes or Yams

(Packed without sugar syrup)

Refer to footnotes for special dietary information

INGREDIENTS	WEIGHTS/MEASURES	YIELD ADJUST.	METHOD
Canned drained sweet potatoes or yams	2 No. 10 cans or 8 No. 2½ cans or 4 No. 3 cyl. cans		1. Put half of the sweet potatoes or yams in each of 2 buttered steam table pans.
Brown sugar . . . . Water. Salt . . . . Margarine	2½ quarts 1 cup 1 tablespoon 1 cup (8 ounces)		2. Combine sugar, water, salt and margarine; cook and stir over low heat until sugar is dissolved and mixture is smooth. Pour ½ of the syrup over potatoes in each of the pans. 3. Bake 25 minutes or until very hot and lightly browned. Spoon syrup over sweet potatoes or yams a couple of times during the baking period. Serve hot.

YIELD
50 portions (2 pans)

PORTION SIZE
½ cup (2 or 3 pieces)

PAN SIZE
12 × 20 × 2-inch steam table pans

TEMPERATURE
350°F. Oven

DIETARY INFORMATION
May be used as written for general, no added salt, bland, low fat, low cholesterol, soft and mechanical soft diets.

YIELD
50 portions (2 pans)

PORTION SIZE
1/2 cup (2 or 3 pieces)

PAN SIZE
12 × 20 × 2-inch steam table pans

TEMPERATURE
350°F. Oven

DIETARY INFORMATION
May be used as written for general, no added salt, bland, low fat, low cholesterol, soft and mechanical soft diets.

Glazed Sweet Potatoes or Yams
(Packed with sugar syrup)

Refer to footnotes for special dietary information

INGREDIENTS	WEIGHTS/MEASURES	YIELD ADJUST.	METHOD
Sweet potatoes or yams	2½ No. 10 cans or 10 No. 2½ cans or 5 No. 3 cyl. cans		1. Drain sweet potatoes or yams; keep syrup for use in step 2. Put ½ of the sweet potatoes or yams in each of 2 buttered steam table pans.
Sugar	1 quart		2. Combine sugars, salt, cornstarch and syrup; cook and stir over low heat for 5 minutes; add margarine; mix well. Pour ½ of the syrup over sweet potatoes or yams in each pan.
Brown sugar	3 cups		
Salt	1½ tablespoons		3. Bake 30 minutes. Spoon syrup in pan over potatoes every 10 minutes. Serve hot.
Cornstarch	⅓ cup		
Syrup from potatoes and water	1 quart		
Margarine	1 cup (8 ounces)		

Mashed Sweet Potatoes or Yams

(Packed without sugar syrup)

Refer to footnotes for special dietary information

INGREDIENTS	WEIGHTS/MEASURES	YIELD ADJUST.	METHOD
Nonfat dry milk . . . . .½ cup Warm water . . . . .3 cups			1. Stir dry milk into warm water in mixer bowl; mix at low speed until milk is dissolved.
Sweet potatoes or yams . . . . . .1½ No. 10 cans or 6 No. 2½ cans or 3 No. 3 cyl. cans			2. Drain sweet potatoes or yams well; add to milk; beat at low speed until smooth and free from lumps.
Salt .1 tablespoon Margarine . . . . .1 cup (8 ounces) Sugar . . . . .½ cup			3. Add salt, margarine and sugar to sweet potatoes or yams; mix at moderate speed 1 minute or until well blended.

YIELD
50 portions (1 pan)

PORTION SIZE
½ cup (No. 8 dipper)

PAN SIZE
Roasting pan

TEMPERATURE
350°F. Oven

DIETARY INFORMATION
May be used as written for general, no added salt, bland, low cholesterol, soft and mechanical soft diets. Diabetic diets — ⅓ cup serving provides 1 bread and 1 fat exchanges.

YIELD
50 portions (2 pans)

PORTION SIZE
½ cup (2 or 3 pieces)

PAN SIZE
12 × 20 x 2-inch steam table pans

TEMPERATURE
350°F. Oven

DIETARY INFORMATION
May be used as written for general, no added salt, bland, low cholesterol and soft diets.

Yams or Sweet Potatoes with Pineapple

(Packed without sugar syrup)

Refer to footnotes for special dietary information

INGREDIENTS	WEIGHTS/MEASURES	YIELD ADJUST.	METHOD
Yams or sweet potatoes	2 No. 10 cans or 8 No. 2½ cans or 4 No. 3 cyl. cans		1. Drain yams or sweet potatoes well; put half of the yams or sweet potatoes in each of 2 buttered steam table pans.
Drained crushed pineapple . . . Brown sugar . . . . Margarine . . . . Salt	3 quarts (1 No. 10 can) 1 quart 1 cup (8 ounces) 2 teaspoons		2. Put pineapple, sugar, margarine and salt in mixer bowl; mix 1 minute at low speed. Spread ½ of the pineapple mixture evenly over yams or sweet potatoes in each of the 2 pans. 3. Bake 1 hour or until lightly browned and very hot; serve hot.

Au Gratin Potatoes

Refer to footnotes for special dietary information

INGREDIENTS	WEIGHTS/MEASURES	YIELD ADJUST.	METHOD
White thinly sliced fresh potatoes . . . . .12 pounds, 8 ounces Boiling water. . . . . .as necessary Salt . . . . .1 tablespoon			1. Cover potatoes with boiling water; add salt; bring to a boil; cook 10 minutes or until just tender; drain well. 2. Put drained potatoes into steam table pan.
Nonfat dry milk . . . . .1½ quarts Warm water. . . . . .1 gallon			3. Stir dry milk into water; mix well; heat to just below boiling point. Do not boil.
Melted margarine . . . . .1 cup (8 ounces) All-purpose flour . . . . .2 cups Salt . . . . .1 tablespoon Diced or grated cheddar or American process cheese . .2 quarts (2 pounds)			4. Combine melted margarine, flour and salt and stir until smooth; add to hot milk and cook and stir, using a wire whip, over moderate heat until thickened and smooth. Remove sauce from heat; add cheese and stir until smooth and the cheese is melted. Pour sauce over the potatoes and stir lightly to distribute the sauce throughout the potatoes.
Paprika . . . . .2 teaspoons			5. Sprinkle paprika over potatoes and bake, uncovered, about 30 minutes or until potatoes are hot and lightly browned. Serve hot.

YIELD
50 portions (about 1½ gallons)

PORTION SIZE
½ cup (4 ounces)

PAN SIZE
Heavy 3-gallon pot
12 × 20 × 4-inch steam table pan

TEMPERATURE
375°F. Oven

DIETARY INFORMATION
May be used as written for general, no added salt, bland and soft diets.
Diabetic diets — each serving provides 1½ bread, 1 lean meat and 1 fat exchanges.

YIELD
50 portions

PORTION SIZE
1 potato

PAN SIZE
18 × 26-inch sheet pan

TEMPERATURE
400°F. Oven

DIETARY INFORMATION
May be used as written for general, no added salt, low fat, soft and low cholesterol diets. Diabetic diets — each small baked potato provides 1 bread exchange. Bland and mechanical soft diets should be served the baked potato without the skin.

Baked Potatoes

Refer to footnotes for special dietary information

INGREDIENTS	WEIGHTS/MEASURES	YIELD ADJUST.	METHOD
Medium-size white baking potatoes ....50 (about 15 pounds) Paprika ....as necessary			1. Scrub potatoes thoroughly; remove any bad spots and cut the ends off each potato. Place potatoes on a lightly greased sheet pan. 2. Bake 1 hour or until soft when squeezed. Slit the top of each potato crosswise and open slightly. Sprinkle with paprika and serve hot.

Creamed Potatoes

Refer to footnotes for special dietary information

INGREDIENTS	WEIGHTS/MEASURES	YIELD ADJUST.	METHOD
Water.....................2 quarts Chicken soup and gravy base. .¼ cup			1. Heat water to boiling point; add soup and gravy base; mix well to form a hot stock.
All-purpose flour............1 cup Nonfat dry milk.............1½ cups Cold water................1¼ quarts			2. Stir flour and milk into cold water; beat with a whisk or hand beater until smooth; pour slowly into hot stock, stirring constantly. 3. Cook sauce over low heat until thickened, stirring constantly.
Margarine ....1 cup (8 ounces) Salt ....1 tablespoon Pepper..................1 teaspoon			4. Add margarine to hot sauce; stir until smooth; add salt and pepper; cook, stirring constantly, another 2 minutes or until starchy taste is gone.
Canned whole white potatoes .2 No. 10 cans			5. Heat potatoes in their own juice; drain well; discard liquid. Add hot potatoes to sauce; serve hot.

YIELD
50 portions (about 1½ gallons)

PORTION SIZE
½ cup (4 ounces)

PAN SIZE
Heavy 5-gallon pot

NOTE
12 pounds, 8 ounces peeled fresh white potatoes may be cooked and used instead of the canned potatoes in step 5. 14 pounds, 8 ounces fresh white potatoes will yield approximately 12 pounds, 8 ounces peeled white potatoes.

DIETARY INFORMATION
May be used as written for general, no added salt, low fat, low cholesterol and mechanical soft diets. Diabetic diets — each serving provides 1 bread and 1 fat exchanges.

YIELD
50 portions (1 pan)

PORTION SIZE
½ cup (4 ounces)

PAN SIZE
Heavy 5-gallon pot
Roasting pan

TEMPERATURE
450°F. Oven

VARIATIONS
1. Home-fried potatoes: Slice fresh potatoes instead of dicing them; put in hot fat in roasting pan without cooking them; add salt and pepper; bake 25 to 30 minutes or until tender, turning them over about every 10 minutes to be sure they brown evenly.
2. O'Brien potatoes: Cook potatoes as directed in basic recipe. Fry 1 cup of chopped onions and 1 cup chopped fresh green pepper in ½ cup (4 ounces) margarine until onions are golden; add to potatoes about 5 minutes before they are ready to come out of the oven.

NOTES
1. About 1¾ gallons chopped or diced, cooked cold white potatoes may be used instead of cooking raw potatoes in step 1. 2. 14 pounds, 8 ounces fresh white potatoes will yield approximately 12 pounds, 8 ounces peeled potatoes.

DIETARY INFORMATION
May be used as written for general, no added salt, low cholesterol and low fat diets. Diabetic diets — each serving provides 1 bread and 1 fat exchanges. Bland diets — omit pepper.

Hashed Brown Potatoes

Refer to footnotes for special dietary information

INGREDIENTS	WEIGHTS/MEASURES	YIELD ADJUST.	METHOD
Fresh diced white potatoes . . .12 pounds, 8 ounces Boiling water. . . . . .to cover Salt . . . . .3 tablespoons			1. Cover potatoes with boiling water; add salt; simmer 15 to 20 minutes or until tender; drain well.
Margarine . . . . .1 cup (8 ounces) Salt . . . . .1 tablespoon Pepper. . . . . .1 teaspoon			2. Heat margarine in roasting pan. Put diced potatoes in pan; sprinkle with salt and pepper. 3. Bake 20 to 25 minutes, stirring about every 5 minutes, until potatoes are browned.

Mashed Potatoes

Refer to footnotes for special dietary information

INGREDIENTS	WEIGHTS/MEASURES	YIELD ADJUST.	METHOD
Fresh white potatoes peeled and quartered . . . . .12 pounds, 8 ounces Boiling water. . . . . .to cover Salt . . . . .2 tablespoons			1. Cover potatoes with water; add salt; bring to a boil; reduce heat; simmer 20 minutes or until tender; drain well. Put into a mixer bowl; beat at slow speed until broken up.
Salt . . . . .2 tablespoons Margarine . . . . .1 cup (8 ounces)			2. Add salt and margarine to potatoes; beat at high speed 3 to 5 minutes or until smooth and fluffy.
Nonfat dry milk. . . . . .1½ cups Warm water. . . . . .2 cups			3. Stir milk into warm water; add to potatoes; beat 2 more minutes or until light and fluffy; serve hot.

YIELD
50 portions (about 1½ gallons)

PORTION SIZE
½ cup (No. 8 dipper)

PAN SIZE
Heavy 5-gallon pot

VARIATION
Hot mashed potato salad: Use 1 cup water instead of 2 cups water in step 3. Add 2 cups salad dressing, 1½ cups finely chopped onions, 10 chopped hard-cooked eggs, 1 cup finely chopped green peppers and ½ cup finely chopped pimiento to mashed potatoes after step 3. Serve warm.

NOTES
14 pounds, 8 ounces fresh white potatoes will yield approximately 12 pounds, 8 ounces peeled potatoes.

DIETARY INFORMATION
May be used as written for general, no added salt, bland, low fat, low cholesterol, soft and mechanical soft diets. Diabetic diets — each serving yields 1 bread exchange.

Oven-Browned Potatoes

Refer to footnotes for special dietary information

YIELD
50 portions (1 pan)

PORTION SIZE
1 medium potato

PAN SIZE
Roasting pan

TEMPERATURE
425°F. Oven

NOTES
1. 14 pounds, 8 ounces fresh white potatoes will yield approximately 12 pounds, 8 ounces peeled potatoes.
2. Potatoes may be boiled 10 minutes and drained before baking to shorten baking time.

DIETARY INFORMATION
May be used as written for general, no added salt and soft diets. Diabetic diets — each serving of one small potato yields 1 bread and 1 fat exchanges. Bland diets — omit pepper.

INGREDIENTS	WEIGHTS/MEASURES	YIELD ADJUST.	METHOD
Fresh white potatoes peeled and cut in halves or quarters	12 pounds, 8 ounces		1. Put potatoes in well-greased baking pan.
Margarine, melted.	1 cup (8 ounces)		2. Pour margarine over potatoes; sprinkle with salt, pepper and paprika.
Salt	1 tablespoon		3. Bake 1½ hours or until browned and tender; turn potatoes twice during the baking period.
Pepper.	1 teaspoon		
Paprika	1½ tablespoons		

Paprika Buttered Potatoes

Refer to footnotes for special dietary information

INGREDIENTS	WEIGHTS/MEASURES	YIELD ADJUST.	METHOD
Fresh white peeled potatoes . .12 pounds, 8 ounces Boiling water. . . . . .as necessary Salt .3 tablespoons			1. Cover potatoes with water; add salt; simmer about 20 minutes or until tender; drain well; keep ½ cup potato water for use in step 2.
Margarine, melted. . . . . .1 cup (8 ounces) Hot potato water. . . . . .½ cup Paprika . . . . .2 tablespoons			2. Mix margarine with hot potato water; mix well; pour over hot potatoes. 3. Sprinkle paprika lightly over each serving of potatoes.

YIELD
50 portions

PORTION SIZE
1 medium potato

PAN SIZE
Heavy 5-gallon pot

VARIATIONS
1. Parsley buttered potatoes: Omit paprika in step 3; use chopped fresh parsley to sprinkle over potatoes.
2. Polish potatoes and onions: Cook potatoes as directed above in step 1 but do not follow steps 2 or 3. Fry 3 quarts chopped onions in 1 cup butter or margarine until onions are golden. Chop hot potatoes lightly; garnish each serving of potatoes with some of the fried onions.

NOTE
14 pounds, 8 ounces fresh white potatoes will yield approximately 12 pounds, 8 ounces peeled potatoes.

DIETARY INFORMATION
May be used as written for general, no added salt, low fat, low cholesterol, bland and soft diets. Diabetic diets — each serving provides 1 bread and 1 fat exchanges.

YIELD
50 portions (about 1½ gallons)

PORTION SIZE
½ cup

PAN SIZE
Heavy 5-gallon pot
12 × 20 × 4-inch steam table pan

TEMPERATURE
350°F. Oven

NOTE
14 pounds, 8 ounces fresh white potatoes will yield approximately 12 pounds, 8 ounces peeled potatoes.

DIETARY INFORMATION
May be used as written for general, no added salt, soft, low cholesterol and low fat diets. Diabetic diets — each serving provides 1 bread and 1 lowfat milk exchanges.

Scalloped Potatoes

Refer to footnotes for special dietary information

INGREDIENTS	WEIGHTS/MEASURES	YIELD ADJUST.	METHOD
Fresh white thinly sliced potatoes Boiling water Salt	12 pounds, 8 ounces as necessary 1 tablespoon		1. Cover potatoes with boiling water; add salt; bring to a boil; cook 10 minutes or until barely tender. Drain well. 2. Put drained potatoes into well-greased steam table pan.
Nonfat dry milk Warm water	2 quarts 1¼ gallons		3. Stir dry milk into water; mix well; heat to just below boiling point but do not let boil.
Margarine, melted All-purpose flour Salt Pepper Paprika	1 cup (8 ounces) 1½ cups 1½ tablespoons ½ teaspoon as necessary		4. Mix melted margarine with flour, salt and pepper; add to the hot milk while beating with a wire whip. Cook and stir over low heat until smooth and thickened. 5. Pour sauce over potatoes; stir lightly to mix the potatoes and sauce together. Sprinkle lightly with paprika. Bake 1 hour or until hot and lightly browned.

Spaghetti

Refer to footnotes for special dietary information

INGREDIENTS	WEIGHTS/MEASURES	YIELD ADJUST.	METHOD
Spaghetti . . . . .6 pounds Hot water . . . . .4 gallons Salt . . . . .¼ cup Vegetable oil . . . . .2 tablespoons			1. Stir spaghetti into boiling salted water; add oil; cook about 15 minutes or until tender, stirring occasionally. 2. Drain well; serve hot. If spaghetti is not to be used immediately, it should be covered with cold water and refrigerated or kept in a very cool place. When spaghetti is to be served, it can be put in a wire basket or colander and dipped into boiling water about 2 minutes or until hot. Drain well; serve hot.

YIELD
50 portions (about 3¼ gallons)

PORTION SIZE
1 cup (6 ounces)

PAN SIZE
Heavy 5-gallon pot

DIETARY INFORMATION
May be used as written for general, no added salt, bland, low fat, low cholesterol, soft, mechanical soft and restricted residue diets. Diabetic diets — each serving provides 2 bread exchanges.

Italian Rice (Risotto)

Refer to footnotes for special dietary information

YIELD
50 portions (about 1½ gallons)

PORTION SIZE
½ cup

PAN SIZE
Heavy 3-gallon pot

NOTE
Risotto made with chicken broth is usually served with chicken. It may be made with beef broth and served with beef, if desired.

DIETARY INFORMATION
May be used as written for general, no added salt, bland, low fat, low cholesterol and mechanical soft diets. Diabetic diets — each serving, without the Parmesan cheese, yields 1⅓ bread exchanges.

INGREDIENTS	WEIGHTS/MEASURES	YIELD ADJUST.	METHOD
Finely chopped onions . . . . . . .1 cup Margarine . . . . .½ cup (4 ounces) Long grain rice . . . . .1½ quarts (2 pounds, 12 ounces) Saffron (optional) . . . . .⅛ teaspoon			1. Fry onions in margarine until golden; add rice and saffron; continue to cook and stir about 4 minutes longer or until rice glistens and is golden.
Simmering fat-free chicken broth . . . . .1½ gallons Salt . . . . .as necessary Grated Parmesan cheese (optional) . . . . .3 cups			2. Add 1 quart hot broth to rice, simmer, stirring frequently, for a total of 26 minutes. Add more hot broth to the rice, 1 quart at a time, until all of the broth has been used and absorbed by the rice. Add more salt, if necessary. (The amount of salt needed will depend upon the saltiness of the chicken broth.) 3. Serve hot, sprinkled with Parmesan cheese, using about 1 tablespoon cheese per serving.

Spanish Rice

Refer to footnotes for special dietary information

INGREDIENTS	WEIGHTS/MEASURES	YIELD ADJUST.	METHOD
Chopped bacon . . . . .1 pound, 8 ounces Long grain rice . . . . .1¼ quarts (2 pounds, 4 ounces)			1. Fry bacon until fat is transparent; add rice and fry, stirring constantly, for 2 to 3 minutes. Drain off as much fat as possible.
Chopped onions . . . . .3 cups Chopped fresh green peppers .1½ cups Chopped celery. . . . . .3 cups			2. Add onions, fresh green peppers and celery to bacon and rice; cook and stir 2 to 3 minutes longer.
Salt . . . . .1 tablespoon Pepper. . . . . .½ teaspoon Tomato puree . . . . .1¼ quarts Hot beef stock . . . . .2 quarts Sugar. . . . . .2 tablespoons Garlic granules . . . . .1 teaspoon			3. Add salt, pepper, tomato puree, beef stock, sugar and garlic to rice mixture; cook and stir over medium heat for 5 minutes; pour into deep steam table pan; cover tightly with aluminum foil; bake 1 hour or until rice is tender.

YIELD
50 portions (about 1½ gallons)

PORTION SIZE
½ cup (No. 8 dipper)

PAN SIZE
12 × 20 × 4-inch steam table pan

TEMPERATURE
350°F. Oven

DIETARY INFORMATION
May be used as written for general, no added salt and low fat diets. Diabetic diets — each serving provides 1½ bread exchanges. Bland diets — omit pepper. Low cholesterol diets — omit bacon in step 1. Fry rice in ¼ cup vegetable oil.

YIELD
50 portions (about 1½ gallons)

PORTION SIZE
½ cup

PAN SIZE
12 × 20 × 4-inch steam table pan

TEMPERATURE
350°F. Oven

DIETARY INFORMATION
May be used as written for general, no added salt, bland, low fat, low cholesterol, soft and mechanical soft diets. Diabetic diets — each serving provides 1 bread exchange.

Oven-Baked Rice

Refer to footnotes for special dietary information

INGREDIENTS WEIGHTS/MEASURES	YIELD ADJUST.	METHOD
Long grain rice . . . . .1½ quarts (2 pounds, 12 ounces) Hot water, fat-free chicken or beef broth . . . . .3 quarts Salt . . . . .1 tablespoon		1. Place rice, hot water or broth and salt in steam table pan. (The salt will not be necessary if salted broth is used.) Cover tightly with aluminum foil and bake 30 to 35 minutes or until rice is tender. 2. Uncover the rice; stir lightly with a fork and allow it to fluff and dry, covered with a clean cloth, for about 5 minutes.

Chapter 9
Salads

Information
166

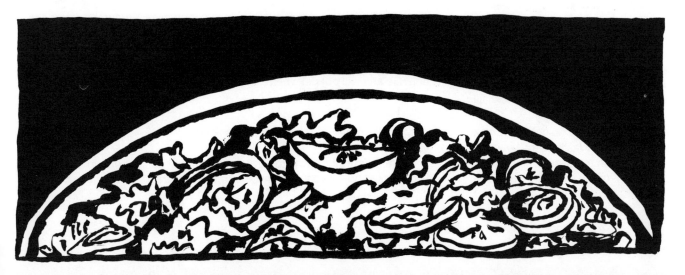

Salad Information

Salads are a very important part of the diet in nursing/convalescent homes and hospitals. They add color, texture, taste and good nutrition to the diet and should always be emphasized in any diet which allows their use.

Because there are so many residents with diabetes these days, a special effort has been made to adapt recipes whenever possible for use in the diabetic diet. diabetic gelatins and dressings are widely available and add much to the diabetic diet. Diabetic dressings can also be prepared in the facility using dressing recipes at the end of this chapter.

Since it is widely recognized that fiber is important in the diet of almost everyone and particularly in the diet of nursing home residents, high-fiber recipes have been included whenever possible.

SALAD GREENS

1. An attractive tossed vegetable salad begins with clean, crisp, cold greens. Greens wilt from day to day even when kept under proper refrigeration. All salad greens are fragile and must be treated gently at all times. Do not trim or wash greens, or remove them from their shipping containers unless they are to be used within 24 hours. Wash and trim greens as soon as possible after you remove them from their shipping container. Do not allow greens to stand at room temperature any longer than necessary. They should be kept refrigerated until they are ready to be cleaned and then put back into the refrigerator after they are cleaned until they are to be used.

2. Cleaning salad greens:

a. Discard any damaged outer leaves but keep as many of the outer leaves as possible for color and because they are richer in vitamins than the inner paler leaves. If the greens are wilted, they can be crisped in cold water. Separate leaves of romaine or escarole, remove the stems and discard the stems. Leave lettuce whole except for removing the core.

b. Fill a sink ⅔ full of lukewarm or cool water; add some salt to get rid of any insects and put the whole head of lettuce with the core removed or the separated leaves of other greens in the water. If 2 sinks are available, fill the second sink ⅔ full of cold water.

c. Soak greens in the first sink for about 15 minutes; do not fill the sink too full of greens because they need plenty of room. Wash greens by lifting them up and down in the sink and then put them in the second sink. Never leave the greens in the sink and let the water out of the sink. The water and any dirt or insects should be left in the sink and the greens removed from the water.

d. Greens should soak in the second sink for another 15 minutes and then be lifted up and down to wash them. They should be drained in a large colander or rack on the drain board. Drain greens well but leave a little bit of water clinging to the leaves to help keep the greens crisp. Refrigerate the clean greens for an hour or so before they are used to crisp them. A big plastic bag is good to store them or they can be piled lightly in a steam table pan and kept lightly covered in the refrigerator. A damp cloth or plastic may be put over them during storage.

3. Salad greens should not be cut with a knife; they should be torn into convenient bite-size pieces unless the lettuce is to be shredded in which case it is necessary to use a knife.

4. Do not add the salad dressing to the greens until just before they are to be served.

GELATIN SALADS

1. Gelatin salads should always be served chilled on cold dishes and should not be allowed to stand in a warm room.

2. Fruit-flavored gelatin must be thoroughly dissolved in boiling hot water before cold water or cold fruit juice is added to the gelatin. Never use more liquid than the recipe includes because if too much liquid is used, the gelatin will not harden. Never use less liquid than the recipe includes because if not enough liquid is used, the gelatin will be rubbery and tough.

3. Fruits will be more evenly distributed throughout the gelatin if the fruit is not added to the gelatin until it is partially firm.

4. Diabetic gelatin should be made from diabetic fruit-flavored gelatin and diabetic fruits or vegetables such as cabbage and cucumbers or it can be made with plain gelatin with lemon juice for flavor and diabetic fruits or vegetables.

Note: In gelatin recipes which call for pineapple, use canned pineapple only. Gelatin will not gel when fresh pineapple is used.

FRUIT SALADS

1. Fruit salads should always be served chilled on cold dishes and should not be allowed to stand in a warm room.

2. Canned fruits for mixed fruit salad should be well drained. The fruit juice should be saved for use in gelatin, as a beverage or for a sauce.

3. Fresh fruits will retain their color and not turn brown if they are dropped into fruit juices with some acid in the juice such as pineapple or orange juice or into water with lemon juice in it while they are being prepared. They should be well drained before they are combined with other ingredients for the salad.

4. Fresh fruits, except for bananas, for salads or other uses should be refrigerated until used.

5. Fresh fruits should be thoroughly washed and drained and any bruised spots removed before they are prepared for use in salads.

6. The use of prepared orange and grapefruit segments for salads is generally more economical than buying the fresh oranges and grapefruit and preparing the segments in the kitchen.

YIELD
50 portions (about 2 gallons)

PORTION SIZE
2/3 cup (No. 6 dipper)

VARIATION
CHICKEN or TURKEY POTATO SALAD:
Add 3 quarts diced, cooked potatoes in
step 2. Use 1½ quarts salad dressing
and 2 tablespoons salt instead of the
amounts shown. A ¾ cup serving of
chicken or turkey potato salad will yield
2 ounces of cooked meat and ¼ cup
potatoes.

DIETARY INFORMATION
May be used as written for general and
bland diets. Diabetic diets — substitute
cooked diabetic salad dressing for
dressing in step 2. Each serving, using
cooked diabetic salad dressing,
provides ½ bread and 2 lean meat
exchanges. No added salt diets — omit
pickles or pickle relish. Each serving
provides 2 ounces cooked chicken and
eggs.

Chicken or Turkey Salad

Refer to footnotes for special dietary information

INGREDIENTS WEIGHTS/MEASURES	YIELD ADJUST.	METHOD
Cold cooked chicken or turkey, cut in ½-inch cubes . . . . . . .5 pounds, 4 ounces Salad dressing . . . . .1 quart		1. (Trim any fat or gristle and skin from chicken or turkey before it is weighed.) Turkey or chicken rolls or cubed, precooked product may be used instead of cooking fresh poultry if desired. 2. Toss chicken or turkey with salad dressing until pieces of poultry are coated with dressing.
Chopped sweet pickles or sweet pickle relish . . . . .2 cups Finely diced celery . . . . .2 quarts Chopped hard-cooked eggs . . .16 Salt . . . . .1 tablespoon		3. Add pickles, celery, eggs and salt to poultry; mix lightly and refrigerate until served.

Ham Salad

Refer to footnotes for special dietary information

INGREDIENTS WEIGHTS/MEASURES	YIELD ADJUST.	METHOD
Salad dressing . . . . .1 quart Finely chopped celery . . . . . . .2 quarts Finely chopped onions. . . . . . .1 cup Chopped pimiento-stuffed green olives. . . . . .1 cup Salad mustard. . . . . .¼ cup Sweet pickle relish . . . . .1 cup		1. Combine salad dressing, celery, onions, olives, mustard and pickle relish in a bowl and mix well.
Coarsely ground cooked ham. .4 pounds, 12 ounces Chopped hard-cooked eggs . . .24		2. Add ham and eggs to salad dressing mixture; mix lightly, cover and refrigerate until served.

YIELD
50 portions (about 1½ gallons)

PORTION SIZE
½ cup (No. 8 dipper)

DIETARY INFORMATION
May be used as written for general and bland diets. Diabetic diets — substitute cooked diabetic salad dressing for dressing in step 1. Each serving, using cooked diabetic salad dressing, provides 1 vegetable, 1 medium fat and 1 fat meat exchanges. No added salt diets — omit olives and pickle relish. Each serving provides 2 ounces ham and eggs.

YIELD
50 portions

PORTION SIZE
2 halves

DIETARY INFORMATION
May be used as written for general, no added salt and bland diets. Diabetic diets — substitute cooked diabetic salad dressing for the dressing in step 2. Each serving, using cooked diabetic salad dressing, provides 1 medium fat meat exchange. Each serving provides 1 egg.

Deviled Eggs

Refer to footnotes for special dietary information

INGREDIENTS	WEIGHTS/MEASURES	YIELD ADJUST.	METHOD
Eggs . . . . .50 Cold water. . . . . .as necessary			1. Cover eggs with cold water; bring to a simmer; cook over low heat 10 to 15 minutes. Drain well; cover immediately with cold water. Remove shells and cut eggs lengthwise. Remove yolks to a bowl; arrange the egg whites in rows on a tray.
Hot milk. . . . . .½ cup Salad dressing . . . . .1¼ cups Salt . . . . .1 tablespoon Salad mustard. . . . . .¼ cup Vinegar . . . . .¼ cup Paprika (optional) . . . . .as necessary			2. Mash yolks; add hot milk; mix until well blended; add salad dressing, salt, mustard and vinegar; mix until smooth and well blended. 3. Stuff egg whites with egg yolk mixture using a heaping tablespoon filling for each of the halves. Egg yolks may be dusted with a garnish of paprika if desired.

Egg Salad

Refer to footnotes for special dietary information

INGREDIENTS WEIGHTS/MEASURES	YIELD ADJUST.	METHOD
Finely chopped celery . . . . . . .3 cups Finely chopped sweet pickles .1 cup Finely chopped pimiento . . . . .1 cup Salad mustard. . . . . .¼ cup Salt . . . . .1 tablespoon Salad dressing . . . . .2½ cups		1. Combine celery, pickles, pimiento, mustard, salt and salad dressing; mix well.
Peeled hard-cooked eggs 50		2. Chop eggs; add to salad dressing mixture. Toss lightly; refrigerate until served. (Prepare egg salad as close to serving time as possible.)

YIELD
50 portions (about 1 gallon)

PORTION SIZE
⅓ cup (No. 12 dipper)

DIETARY INFORMATION
May be used as written for general and bland diets. Diabetic diets — substitute cooked diabetic salad dressing for the dressing in step 1. Each serving, using cooked diabetic salad dressing, provides 1 vegetable and 1 medium fat meat exchanges. No added salt diets — omit pickles in step 1. Each serving provides 1 egg.

YIELD
48 portions (2 pans)

PORTION SIZE
1 square (1 whole egg)

PAN SIZE
12 × 20 × 2-inch steam table pans

DIETARY INFORMATION
May be used as written for general and bland diets. Diabetic diets — substitute diabetic fruit-flavored gelatin for gelatin in step 1. Each serving, using diabetic gelatin, provides 1 high fat meat exchange. No added salt diets — omit olives. Each serving provides 1 egg.

Molded Egg Salad

Refer to footnotes for special dietary information

INGREDIENTS	WEIGHTS/MEASURES	YIELD ADJUST.	METHOD
Lemon-flavored gelatin........3 pounds (1¾ quarts) Salt.....................2 tablespoons Boiling water...............1 gallon			1. Dissolve gelatin and salt in boiling water.
Crushed ice...............1 gallon Vinegar...................½ cup			2. Add crushed ice and vinegar to gelatin; mix well and chill, if necessary, until it is syrupy. 3. Pour ¼ inch of syrupy gelatin into each of 2 steam table pans; chill until gelatin is firm.
Deviled eggs..............4 dozen (96 halves)			4. Spoon a small amount of the syrupy gelatin over each of the deviled egg halves, covering yolk lightly with a glaze of gelatin. Chill eggs while gelatin in pans is getting firm; then invert eggs onto gelatin layer; chill together until firm.
Diced celery..............1 quart Chopped pimiento-stuffed green olives.............1½ quarts			5. Combine celery and olives with remaining gelatin; spoon over the eggs; chill until firm. 6. Cut gelatin into squares with 2 egg halves in each square. Turn squares over so that the yellow of eggs will show; serve on lettuce leaf with salad dressing if desired.

Pasta Salad with Salmon

Refer to footnotes for special dietary information

INGREDIENTS	WEIGHTS/MEASURES	YIELD ADJUST.	METHOD
Rotini. . . . . .2 pounds, 8 ounces Boiling water. . . . . .3 gallons Salt .2 tablespoons Vegetable oil . . . . .1 tablespoon			1. Drop rotini in boiling salted water; stir lightly to mix; add oil; cook, uncovered, over medium heat 16 minutes or until tender. Drain rotini well but do not rinse it.
Italian-style vinegar and oil salad dressing . . . . .1 quart			2. Pour salad dressing over hot rotini; toss dressing and rotini together until each piece is coated with dressing; cool to lukewarm.
Chopped salad-style pimiento-stuffed green olives . . . . . . .2 cups Finely chopped onion. . . . . . . .1 cup Chopped hard-cooked eggs . . .24 Salt .1 tablespoon			3. Put olives, onions, hard-cooked eggs and salt on top of rotini in bowl.
Canned salmon. . . . . .6 1-pound cans Cooked peas. . . . . .1 quart			4. Drain salmon; remove skin and bones; flake salmon; add salmon and peas to bowl with rotini and other ingredients; toss lightly. 5. Refrigerate salad until served.

YIELD
50 portions (about 2½ gallons)

PORTION SIZE
¾ cup

NOTES
Rotini is a screw-shaped macaroni product. If it is unavailable, shell macaroni or elbow macaroni may be substituted for the rotini.

DIETARY INFORMATION
May be used as written for general diets. Diabetic diets — substitute cooked diabetic salad dressing for dressing in step 2. Each serving, using cooked diabetic salad dressing, provides 1 bread, 1 vegetable and 2 medium fat meat exchanges. No added salt diets — omit olives. Each serving provides 2 ounces of salmon and eggs.

YIELD
50 portions (about 1½ gallons)

PORTION SIZE
½ cup (No. 8 dipper)

DIETARY INFORMATION
May be used as written for general and bland diets. Diabetic diets — substitute diabetic cooked salad dressing for dressing in step 1. Each serving, using diabetic cooked salad dressing, provides ½ bread, 1 lean meat and 1 fat exchanges. No added salt diets — omit sweet relish. Each serving provides 1 ounce of cheese and eggs.

Peas and Cheese Salad

Refer to footnotes for special dietary information

INGREDIENTS	WEIGHTS/MEASURES	YIELD ADJUST.	METHOD
Salad dressing . . . . .3 cups Finely chopped onions . . . . . . .1 cup Chopped celery. . . . . .2 cups Sweet pickle relish . . . . .2 cups Chopped pimiento . . . . .¼ cup Salt . . . . .1 tablespoon Cubed cheddar or American process cheese. . . . . .2 pounds			1. Combine salad dressing, onions, celery, pickle relish, pimiento and salt in a large mixing bowl; stir to blend well; add cheese; mix well.
Chopped hard-cooked eggs . . .18 Drained canned peas . . . . .3 quarts (1 No. 10 can)			2. Add eggs and peas to salad dressing mixture; mix lightly, cover and refrigerate until served.

Tunafish Salad

Refer to footnotes for special dietary information

INGREDIENTS	WEIGHTS/MEASURES	YIELD ADJUST.	METHOD
Salad dressing . . . . .1 quart Sweet pickle relish . . . . .1½ cups Finely chopped celery . . . . . . .2½ quarts Finely chopped onions. . . . . . .1 cup Salt . . . . .1 tablespoon			1. Combine salad dressing, pickle relish, celery, onions and salt in a large mixing bowl; stir to mix well.
Drained flaked tunafish . . . . . .4 pounds, 12 ounces Chopped hard-cooked eggs . . .24			2. Add tunafish and eggs to salad dressing mixture; mix lightly, cover and refrigerate until served.

VARIATION
SALMON SALAD: Substitute 6 1-pound cans of salmon for tunafish in step 2. Drain salmon, discard the juice, skin and bones; break the salmon into smaller pieces and add with the eggs to salad dressing mixture.

DIETARY INFORMATION
May be used as written for general and bland diets. Diabetic diets — substitute cooked diabetic salad dressing for dressing in step 1. Each serving, using cooked diabetic salad dressing, provides 1 vegetable and 2 lean meat exchanges. No added salt diets — omit pickle relish in step 1. Each serving provides 2 ounces tunafish and eggs.

YIELD
50 portions (about 1½ gallons)

PORTION SIZE
½ cup (No. 8 dipper)

DIETARY INFORMATION
May be used as written for general and bland diets. Diabetic diets — substitute diabetic cooked salad dressing for dressing in step 2. Each serving, using cooked diabetic salad dressing, provides 1½ bread and 1 medium fat exchanges for ½ cup serving and 1 bread and 1 medium fat meat exchanges for ⅓ cup serving. No added salt diets — omit olives and pickle relish. Each serving provides 1 ounce cheese and eggs.

Macaroni Salad

Refer to footnotes for special dietary information

INGREDIENTS WEIGHTS/MEASURES	YIELD ADJUST.	METHOD
Macaroni. . . . . .3 pounds (3 quarts) Salt . . . . .2 tablespoons Boiling water. . . . . .3 gallons Vegetable oil . . . . .1 tablespoon		1. Drop macaroni in boiling salted water; stir lightly to mix; add oil; cook, uncovered, over medium heat 10 to 12 minutes or until tender. Drain well.

Salad dressing . . . . .1 quart
Salt . . . . .1 tablespoon
Diced or shredded American
   process cheese. . . . . .1 pound, 8 ounces
Chopped salad-style pimiento-
   stuffed green olives . . . . . . .1½ cups
Sweet pickle relish . . . . .1½ cups
Finely chopped celery . . . . . . .1 quart
Chopped hard-cooked eggs . . .26
		2. Put salad dressing and salt in bottom of a large mixing bowl; add cheese, olives, relish, celery and eggs; mix lightly but thoroughly.
		3. Add macaroni to salad dressing mixture; mix lightly but thoroughly; cover and refrigerate until served.

Pasta Salad

Refer to footnotes for special dietary information

INGREDIENTS WEIGHTS/MEASURES	YIELD ADJUST.	METHOD

Rotini, shells, elbow macaroni
   or other shapes of pasta. . . .1 pound
Italian or French-style vinegar
   and oil dressing . . . . .2 cups
		1. Cook pasta according to directions on the package; drain well.
		2. Add salad dressing to the pasta after it is well drained but still hot; toss well to coat the pasta with the dressing; set aside at room temperature to marinate for ½ hour and then mix with vegetables and refrigerate until served.

Peeled cored and well drained
   chopped fresh tomatoes . . .1½ quarts
                (about 2
                pounds)
Chopped onions . . . . .1 cup
Chopped fresh green peppers .1 cup
Thinly sliced celery . . . . .1 cup
		3. Add tomatoes, onions, green peppers and celery to pasta; mix lightly and serve chilled. (Salad should be prepared as close to serving time as possible.)

YIELD
32 portions (1 gallon)

PORTION SIZE
½ cup

NOTE
Various other cooked and/or raw vegetables may be used such as 1½ quarts cooked, chopped broccoli with 1 cup chopped onions and 2 cups chopped, drained fresh tomatoes, using the same proportion of pasta and vegetables as in the basic recipe.

DIETARY INFORMATION
May be used as written for general, no added salt and low cholesterol diets. Diabetic diets — substitute cooked diabetic salad dressing for dressing in step 2. Using diabetic dressing, each serving provides ½ bread exchange.

Apple and Pineapple Salad

Refer to footnotes for special dietary information

YIELD
50 portions (about 1½ gallons)

PORTION SIZE
½ cup

VARIATIONS
1. APPLE, PINEAPPLE and CARROT SALAD: Use 1 quart shredded carrots instead of the celery in step 2.
2. APPLE and RAISIN SALAD: Increase the celery to 2 quarts and use 1 quart raisins instead of the pineapple in step 2.

DIETARY INFORMATION
May be used as written for general, no added salt and bland diets. Diabetic diets — use diabetic cooked salad dressing and pineapple canned without sugar. Each serving, using diabetic cooked salad dressing and pineapple canned without sugar, provides ⅔ fruit exchange.

INGREDIENTS	WEIGHTS/MEASURES	YIELD ADJUST.	METHOD
Fresh apples . . . . .5 pounds Salad dressing . . . . .2 cups			1. Wash apples but don't peel them. Cut apples in quarters, remove core and slice into thin slices; add slices immediately to salad dressing; mix lightly to coat with salad dressing to prevent the slices darkening.
Finely chopped celery . . . . . . .1 quart Drained canned pineapple tidbits . . . . .2 quarts			2. Stir celery and pineapple into apple mixture; mix lightly; refrigerate until served.

Cabbage, Apple and Raisin Salad

Refer to footnotes for special dietary information

INGREDIENTS	WEIGHTS/MEASURES	YIELD ADJUST.	METHOD
Salad dressing . . . . .2 cups Sugar. . . . . .½ cup Salt . . . . .2 teaspoons			1. Mix salad dressing, sugar and salt together in a large mixing bowl.
Cored diced fresh eating apples . . . . .2 quarts			2. Add apples to salad dressing as soon as they are diced; mix lightly to coat each piece with salad dressing to prevent its darkening.
Shredded cabbage . . . . .5 pounds (about 2½ gallons) Washed and drained raisins . . .3 cups (1 pound)			3. Add cabbage and raisins to apples; mix well; cover and refrigerate until served.

YIELD
50 portions (about 1½ gallons)
PORTION SIZE
½ cup

NOTE
6 pounds, 4 ounces cabbage, as purchased, will yield about 5 pounds cleaned, cored and shredded cabbage.

DIETARY INFORMATION
May be used as written for general, no added salt and bland diets. Diabetic diets — omit sugar and use diabetic dressing. Each serving using sugar substitute and diabetic dressing provides 1 fruit exchange.

YIELD
50 portions (about 1½ gallons)

PORTION SIZE
½ cup (No. 8 dipper)

NOTE
6 pounds, 4 ounces cabbage, as purchased, will yield about 5 pounds cleaned and cored cabbage.

DIETARY INFORMATION
May be used as written for general, no added salt and bland diets. Diabetic diets — omit sugar and substitute cooked diabetic salad dressing for dressing in step 1. Use pineapple canned without sugar in step 2. Each serving using sugar substitute, cooked diabetic salad dressing and sugar-free pineapple provides 1 fruit exchange.

Cabbage, Pineapple and Marshmallow Salad

Refer to footnotes for special dietary information

INGREDIENTS	WEIGHTS/MEASURES	YIELD ADJUST.	METHOD
Salad dressing . . . . .2 cups Salt . . . . .2 teaspoons Sugar. . . . . .½ cup			1. Mix salad dressing, salt and sugar together in a large mixing bowl.
Drained crushed pineapple . . .1 quart Miniature marshmallows . . . . .9 cups (1 pound)			2. Add pineapple and marshmallows to salad dressing; stir to mix well.
Shredded cabbage . . . . .5 pounds (about 2½ gallons)			3. Add cabbage to pineapple mixture; mix well; cover and refrigerate until served.

Cranberry and Pineapple Gelatin

Refer to footnotes for special dietary information

INGREDIENTS	WEIGHTS/MEASURES	YIELD ADJUST.	METHOD
Canned jellied cranberry sauce	1 quart (1/3 No. 10 can)		1. Mix cranberry sauce with spoon until it is broken up.
Cherry-flavored gelatin . . . . 1 pound (2 1/3 cups) Boiling water. . . . . 1 quart			2. Dissolve gelatin in boiling water; add cranberry sauce; mix well.
Cold water. . . . . 1 1/4 quarts Lemon juice . . . . 1/3 cup			3. Add cold water and lemon juice to hot gelatin mixture; mix well; pour into a steam table pan; refrigerate until slightly thickened.
Crushed pineapple and juice . . 1 quart Chopped English walnuts . . . . 1 cup (4 ounces)			4. Add pineapple and nuts to gelatin. Stir to mix pineapple and nuts into gelatin; refrigerate until firm.

YIELD
1 pan

PAN SIZE
12 × 20 × 2-inch steam table pan

DIETARY INFORMATION
May be used as written for general, no added salt and bland diets. Diabetic diets — omit sugar, use diabetic fruit-flavored gelatin, fresh cooked cranberries prepared with sugar substitute and sugar-free pineapple and juice. Each serving using sugar substitute, diabetic gelatin and sugar-free pineapple and juice provides 1 vegetable exchange, if the pan is cut 4 × 8. Low fat, soft and mechanical soft diets — omit nuts.

50 portions (about 1½ gallons)

PORTION SIZE
½ cup (No. 8 dipper)

DIETARY INFORMATION
May be used as written for general, no added salt, bland and soft diets. Diabetic diets — use fruit cocktail canned without sugar. Each serving, using sugar-free fruit cocktail, provides 1 bread exchange. Low fat and low cholesterol diets — omit salad dressing.

Mixed Fruit Salad

Refer to footnotes for special dietary information

INGREDIENTS	WEIGHTS/MEASURES	YIELD ADJUST.	METHOD
Canned fruit cocktail ....3 quarts (1 No. 10 can) Fresh bananas ....7 pounds			1. Drain fruit cocktail; save juice for use in step 2. 2. Peel bananas; slice into fruit cocktail juice. Refrigerate both bananas and drained fruit cocktail.
Lettuce ....2 to 3 heads Salad dressing (optional) .....as necessary			3. Trim, wash and drain lettuce. Separate lettuce into leaves; arrange a lettuce leaf on each salad plate or on sheet pans. 4. Just before serving, drain bananas well. Mix drained bananas with drained fruit cocktail; mix lightly. 5. Put a scoop of salad on each lettuce leaf; garnish with salad dressing, if desired.

Molded Applesauce Gelatin

Refer to footnotes for special dietary information

INGREDIENTS	WEIGHTS/MEASURES	YIELD ADJUST.	METHOD
Lemon-flavored gelatin . . . . 1 pound, 8 ounces (3½ cups) Boiling water . . . . 2 quarts			1. Dissolve gelatin in boiling water; refrigerate until slightly thickened.
Canned applesauce . . . . 3 quarts (1 No. 10 can)			2. Stir applesauce into slightly thickened gelatin; mix well. 3. Pour gelatin mixture into steam table pan; refrigerate until firm.

YIELD
1 pan

PAN SIZE
12 × 20 × 2-inch steam table pan

VARIATIONS
1. MOLDED CHERRY APPLESAUCE GELATIN: Substitute hot maraschino cherry juice for the water in step 1. Add 1 cup chopped maraschino cherries with the applesauce in step 2.
2. MOLDED CINNAMON APPLESAUCE GELATIN: Add 1 teaspoon red food coloring to the gelatin in step 1 and add 2 teaspoons ground cinnamon to the applesauce in step 2.

DIETARY INFORMATION
May be used as written for general, no added salt, low fat, low cholesterol, bland, soft and mechanical soft diets. Diabetic diets — use diabetic fruit-flavored gelatin and applesauce canned without sugar. Each serving, using diabetic gelatin and applesauce canned without sugar, provides ⅔ fruit exchange if the pan of gelatin is cut 4 × 8.

YIELD
1 pan

PAN SIZE
12 × 20 × 2-inch steam table pan

DIETARY INFORMATION
May be used as written for general, no added salt and bland diets. Diabetic diets — use diabetic fruit-flavored gelatin and pineapple canned without sugar. Each serving, using diabetic gelatin and pineapple canned without sugar, provides ½ bread exchange, if the pan is cut 4 × 8. Low cholesterol diets — use evaporated skim milk in step 3.

Golden Glow Salad

Refer to footnotes for special dietary information

INGREDIENTS	WEIGHTS/MEASURES	YIELD ADJUST.	METHOD
Crushed pineapple	1½ quarts (½ No. 10 can)		1. Drain pineapple; keep 1½ cups juice for use in step 3.
Lemon-flavored gelatin . . . . Boiling water	1 pound, 4 ounces (3 cups) 1¼ quarts		2. Dissolve gelatin in boiling water; cool to lukewarm.
Evaporated milk . . . . Vinegar . . . . Pineapple juice	1¼ quarts ¾ cup 1½ cups		3. Stirring constantly, add milk, vinegar and then pineapple juice to gelatin; refrigerate until slightly thickened.
Shredded carrots . . . . Shredded cabbage	1 quart 1 quart		4. Add cabbage, carrots and pineapple to slightly thickened gelatin; pour into steam table pan; refrigerate until firm.

Molded Pear and Cottage Cheese Salad

Refer to footnotes for special dietary information

INGREDIENTS	WEIGHTS/MEASURES	YIELD ADJUST.	METHOD
Lime-flavored gelatin . . . . .1 pound (2⅓ cups) Boiling water. . . . . .1 quart Cold water. . . . . .1 quart			1. Dissolve gelatin in boiling water; add cold water; refrigerate until slightly thickened.
Pureed pears. . . . . .1 quart Drained creamed cottage cheese . . . . .2 pounds (1 quart) Finely chopped pimiento . . . . .½ cup			2. Stir pears, cottage cheese and pimiento into slightly thickened gelatin; mix well. 3. Pour gelatin mixture into steam table pan; refrigerate until firm.

YIELD
1 pan

PAN SIZE
12 × 20 × 2-inch steam table pan

DIETARY INFORMATION
May be used as written for general, no added salt, bland, low fat, soft and mechanical soft diets. Diabetic diets — use diabetic fruit-flavored gelatin and pears canned without sugar. Each serving using diabetic gelatin and pears canned without sugar provides ½ skim milk exchange, if the pan is cut 4 × 8. Low cholesterol diets — drain cottage cheese and rinse with lukewarm water before it is used.

YIELD
1 pan

PAN SIZE
12 × 20 × 2-inch steam table pan

VARIATION
PERFECTION SALAD: Add 2 cups chopped fresh green peppers in step 2.

DIETARY INFORMATION
May be used as written for general, no added salt, bland, low fat and low cholesterol diets. Diabetic diets — use diabetic fruit-flavored gelatin and pineapple canned without sugar. Each serving, using diabetic gelatin and pineapple canned without sugar, provides 1/2 vegetable exchange, if the pan is cut 4 × 8.

Molded Pineapple Carrot Salad

Refer to footnotes for special dietary information

INGREDIENTS	WEIGHTS/MEASURES	YIELD ADJUST.	METHOD
Lemon-flavored gelatin . . . . . . .1 pound (2 1/3 cups) Salt . . . . .1 teaspoon Boiling water . . . . .1 quart Cold water . . . . .1 1/2 quarts Vinegar . . . . .1/3 cup			1. Dissolve gelatin and salt in boiling water; add cold water and vinegar; pour into steam table pan; refrigerate until slightly thickened.
Grated carrots . . . . .3 cups Canned crushed pineapple and juice . . . . .1 quart (1/3 No. 10 can)			2. Add carrots and pineapple to slightly thickened gelatin; stir to mix well; refrigerate until firm.

Molded Spiced Cherry Salad

Refer to footnotes for special dietary information

INGREDIENTS	WEIGHTS/MEASURES	YIELD ADJUST.	METHOD
Canned red sour pitted cherries . . . . .3 quarts (1 No. 10 can)			1. Drain cherries; keep juice for use in step 2.
Cherry juice and water . . . . . . .2 quarts Brown sugar . . . . .1 cup Ground cinnamon. . . . . .1 teaspoon Ground cloves. . . . . .½ teaspoon			2. Add water to cherry juice to equal 2 quarts; add sugar, cinnamon and cloves to cherry juice; bring to a boil; reduce heat; simmer for 5 minutes; remove from heat.
Cherry-flavored gelatin . . . . . . .1 pound (2⅓ cups) Cold water. . . . . .1 quart			3. Dissolve gelatin in hot cherry juice; add cold water; mix well. 4. Pour gelatin into steam table pan; chill until slightly thickened. 5. Add drained cherries to slightly thickened gelatin; stir to distribute cherries evenly; chill until firm.

YIELD
1 pan

PAN SIZE
12 × 20 × 2-inch steam table pan

DIETARY INFORMATION
May be used as written for general, no added salt, low fat, low cholesterol and soft diets. Diabetic diets — omit sugar, use diabetic fruit-flavored gelatin and cherries canned without sugar. Each serving, using sugar substitute, diabetic gelatin and cherries canned without sugar, provides ⅔ fruit exchange, if the pan is cut 4 × 8. Bland diets — omit cloves.

YIELD
50 pounds

PORTION SIZE
1 peach half
1/4 cup cottage cheese

VARIATIONS
1. Fruit cocktail and cottage cheese salad: Substitute 1/4 cup of drained, canned fruit cocktail for each peach half in step 2. Arrange the fruit cocktail around the cottage cheese on the lettuce leaf.
2. Pear and cottage cheese salad: Substitute 50 pear halves for the 50 peach halves in step 2.
3. Pineapple and cottage cheese salad: Substitute 50 pineapple slices for the 50 peach halves in step 2.

DIETARY INFORMATION
May be used as written for general, no added salt, bland, low fat and soft diets. Diabetic diets — use peach halves canned without sugar. Each serving, using sugar-free peach halves, provides 1 vegetable and 1 lean meat exchanges. Low cholesterol diets — drain cottage cheese very well or use cottage cheese with skim milk. Each serving provides the equivalent of 1 ounce of cooked meat.

Peach and Cottage Cheese Salad

Refer to footnotes for special dietary information

INGREDIENTS	WEIGHTS/MEASURES	YIELD ADJUST.	METHOD
Lettuce	2 to 3 heads		1. Trim, wash and drain lettuce. Separate lettuce into leaves; arrange a lettuce leaf on each salad plate or on sheet pans.
Canned drained peach halves	50		2. Put a peach half on each lettuce leaf.
Cottage cheese	6 pounds, 8 ounces (3½ quarts)		3. Fill center of each peach half with a No. 16 scoop (¼ cup) of cottage cheese.

Waldorf Salad

Refer to footnotes for special dietary information

YIELD
50 portions (about 1½ gallons)
PORTION SIZE
½ cup

INGREDIENTS	WEIGHTS/MEASURES	YIELD ADJUST.	METHOD
Salad dressing . . . . .2 cups Salt . . . . .2 teaspoons Sugar. . . . . .2 tablespoons			1. Mix salad dressing, salt and sugar in large mixing bowl.
Fresh apples . . . . .5 pounds			2. Wash apples but don't peel them. Cut apples in quarters, remove cores; slice into thin slices; add slices immediately to salad dressing; mix lightly to coat slices with salad dressing to prevent slices darkening.
Finely chopped celery . . . . . . .2 quarts Chopped nuts . . . . .1 quart (1 pound) Miniature marshmallows . . . . .1 quart			3. Stir celery, nuts and marshmallows into apple mixture; mix lightly; refrigerate until served.

DIETARY INFORMATION
May be used as written for general, no added salt and bland diets. Diabetic diets — omit sugar and chopped nuts. Use cooked diabetic salad dressing and increase the chopped celery to 2½ quarts. Each serving with cooked diabetic salad dressing, sugar substitute and with increased celery provides 1 fruit exchange.

YIELD
60 portions (about 2 gallons)

PORTION SIZE
½ cup

PAN SIZE
12-quart stainless steel pot

NOTE
This is a very versatile recipe. Any combination of beans may be used as long as the total amount used totals 6½ quarts. Other vegetables such as julienne carrots, cauliflower and Brussel sprouts may also be included after they have been cooked tender-crisp and well drained.

DIETARY INFORMATION
May be used as written for general, no added salt and low cholesterol diets. Diabetic diets — omit sugar. Add 1½ quarts water to the vinegar in step 1. Cover and simmer 15 minutes and then add sugar substitute to taste after the vinegar mixture is removed from the heat. Each ½ cup serving, using sugar substitute, provides ½ bread exchange. Each ⅓ cup serving, using sugar substitute, provides 1 vegetable exchange. Bland diets — omit fresh green peppers.

Pickled Bean Salad

Refer to footnotes for special dietary information

INGREDIENTS	WEIGHTS/MEASURES	YIELD ADJUST.	METHOD
Vinegar . . . . .1½ quarts Sugar. . . . . .1½ quarts Pickling spices . . . . .⅓ cup			1. Place vinegar, sugar and spices in a stainless steel pot; cover and simmer for 15 minutes. Remove from heat and let set at room temperature overnight; drain well, discarding the spices.

Drained canned green beans . .1½ quarts
Drained canned yellow wax
   beans . . . . .1½ quarts
Drained canned pinto beans . .1 quart
Drained canned baby lima
   beans . . . . .1 quart
Washed and drained canned
   kidney beans. . . . . .1½ quarts
Julienne-cut fresh green
   peppers. . . . . .1 quart
Sliced onions . . . . .1 quart
Sliced or chopped pimientos . .½ cup
			2. Add beans, green peppers, onions and pimientos to vinegar mixture; reheat to simmering but do not let the mixture boil. Remove from heat, cover and let stand at room temperature to cool. Refrigerate at least 24 and preferably 48 hours before the beans are served.

Spiced Beets and Onions

Refer to footnotes for special dietary information

INGREDIENTS	WEIGHTS/MEASURES	YIELD ADJUST.	METHOD
Canned sliced beets.........	1 gallon (1⅓ No. 10 cans)		1. Drain beets well; save liquid to use in step 2.
Beet juice .... Vinegar .... Sugar..................... Mixed pickling spices........ Salt	1 quart 3 cups 3 cups 1 tablespoon 1 tablespoon		2. Combine beet juice, vinegar, sugar, spices and salt. Bring to a boil; simmer 10 minutes; add drained beets; cool to lukewarm.
Thinly sliced onions	1 quart		3. Add onions to beets; cover and refrigerate several hours or overnight. 4. Drain beets and onions well before they are served.

YIELD
50 portions (about 1 gallon)

PORTION SIZE
⅓ cup

DIETARY INFORMATION
May be used as written for general, no added salt and low cholesterol diets. Diabetic diets — omit sugar. Add sugar substitute at the end of step 2. Each serving, using sugar substitute, provides 1 vegetable exchange.

YIELD
50 portions (about 1½ gallons)

PORTION SIZE
½ cup (No. 8 dipper)

VARIATION
Carrot and pineapple salad: Omit the raisins in step 1. Add 1½ quarts drained, canned crushed pineapple to the carrots in step 2.

DIETARY INFORMATION
May be used as written for general, no added salt and bland diets. Diabetic diets — substitute sugar substitute and cooked diabetic salad dressing for sugar and dressing in step 3. Each serving, using sugar substitute and cooked diabetic salad dressing, provides 1 fruit exchange.

Carrot and Raisin Salad

Refer to footnotes for special dietary information

INGREDIENTS	WEIGHTS/MEASURES	YIELD ADJUST.	METHOD
Raisins . . . . .3 cups (1 pound) Hot water . . . . .as necessary			1. Cover raisins with hot water; soak 30 minutes; drain well.
Ground or shredded carrots . . .6 pounds (about 1½ gallons)			2. Combine carrots and raisins; mix lightly.
Salad dressing . . . . .3 cups Milk. . . . . .½ cup Salt . . . . .2 teaspoons Sugar. . . . . .3 tablespoons Vinegar . . . . .2 tablespoons			3. Combine salad dressing, milk, salt, sugar and vinegar; mix well. 4. Add dressing mixture to carrots; toss lightly until vegetables are coated with dressing; cover and refrigerate until used. 5. Toss salad with dressing again just before it is served.

Cole Slaw

Refer to footnotes for special dietary information

INGREDIENTS	WEIGHTS/MEASURES	YIELD ADJUST.	METHOD
Cleaned, cored and shredded cabbage . . . . .6 pounds (about 3 gallons) Shredded carrots . . . . .1 quart Chopped fresh green peppers .1 cup Finely chopped onions . . . . . . .1 cup			1. Put cabbage in a large mixing bowl; add carrots, green peppers and onions; toss lightly.
Sugar. . . . . .3 cups Salt . . . . .1½ tablespoons Vinegar . . . . .3 cups Celery seed . . . . .2 tablespoons			2. Combine sugar, salt, vinegar and celery seed; pour over vegetables; mix lightly but thoroughly. 3. Refrigerate salad 1 to 3 hours. Toss salad with dressing again just before it is served.

YIELD
50 portions (about 1½ gallons)

PORTION SIZE
½ cup (No. 8 dipper)

NOTE
8 pounds cabbage, as purchased, will yield about 6 pounds cleaned and cored cabbage.

DIETARY INFORMATION
May be used as written for general, no added salt and low cholesterol diets. Diabetic diets — omit sugar in step 2. Each serving, using sugar substitute, provides 1 vegetable exchange.

YIELD
50 portions (about 1½ gallons)

PORTION SIZE
½ cup (No. 8 dipper)

VARIATIONS
1. Calico slaw: Use 2 pounds of red cabbage and cut the white cabbage to 4 pounds in step 1. Mix 1 cup chopped pimiento with the salad dressing in step 2.
2. Hamburger slaw: Add 1 quart finely chopped, drained fresh tomatoes and 2 cups finely chopped onions with the other vegetables in step 1. Increase the salt to 3 tablespoons in step 2.
3. Tasty slaw: Add 2 cups finely chopped onions with the other vegetables in step 1.

NOTE
8 pounds of cabbage, as purchased, will yield about 6 pounds cleaned and cored cabbage.

DIETARY INFORMATION
May be used as written for general and no added salt diets. Diabetic diets — omit sugar and substitute cooked diabetic salad dressing for dressing in step 2. Each serving, using sugar substitute and cooked diabetic salad dressing, provides 1 vegetable exchange.

Creamy Cole Slaw

Refer to footnotes for special dietary information

INGREDIENTS	WEIGHTS/MEASURES	YIELD ADJUST.	METHOD
Cleaned cored and shredded cabbage . . . . .6 pounds (about 3 gallons) Shredded carrots . . . . .1½ quarts Chopped fresh green peppers .1½ cups Dehydrated parsley. . . . . .¼ cup			1. Put cabbage in a large mixing bowl; add carrots, fresh green peppers and parsley; toss lightly.
Salad dressing . . . . .2½ cups Sugar. . . . . .1¼ cups Vinegar . . . . .1 cup Salt .2 tablespoons			2. Combine salad dressing, sugar, vinegar and salt; mix well. 3. Pour dressing over vegetables; mix lightly; refrigerate for 2 to 4 hours. Toss salad with dressing again just before it is served.

Molded Cole Slaw

Refer to footnotes for special dietary information

INGREDIENTS	WEIGHTS/MEASURES	YIELD ADJUST.	METHOD
Lemon-flavored gelatin........	1 pound, 8 ounces		1. Dissolve gelatin in hot water; cool to room temperature.
Hot water	3 quarts		2. Combine salad dressing, vinegar and salt; add gelatin gradually to dressing mixture, while beating at low speed. Chill until thickened and then whip, using a whip, at high speed 3 to 4 minutes or until fluffy.
Salad dressing	3 cups		
Vinegar	3/4 cup		
Salt	1 1/2 teaspoons		
Finely chopped cabbage	2 quarts		3. Toss cabbage, green peppers, onions, pimiento and celery seed together to mix well; add to gelatin mixture; mix lightly and pour into pan. Chill until firm and then cut 4 × 8 to serve.
Finely chopped fresh green peppers................	1 cup		
Finely chopped onions.......	1 cup		
Chopped pimientos	3/4 cup		
Celery seed...............	1 tablespoon		

YIELD
32 portions (1 pan)

PORTION SIZE
1 square

PAN SIZE
12 × 20 × 2-inch steam table pan

DIETARY INFORMATION
May be used as written for general and no added salt diets. Diabetic diets — use diabetic fruit-flavored gelatin in step 1 and cooked diabetic salad dressing in step 2. Each serving, using diabetic gelatin and cooked diabetic salad dressing, provides 1 vegetable exchange.

YIELD
50 portions (about 1 gallon)

PORTION SIZE
1/3 cup

VARIATION
Cucumbers in sour cream: Drain the cucumbers well after step 1. Add 2 cups sour cream mixed with 1 tablespoon salt, 1/4 cup sugar and 1/2 cup vinegar instead of the mayonnaise in step 2.

DIETARY INFORMATION
May be used as written for general and no added salt diets. Diabetic diets — substitute cooked diabetic salad dressing for mayonnaise in step 2. Each serving, using cooked diabetic salad dressing, may be considered free.

Cucumber Salad

Refer to footnotes for special dietary information

INGREDIENTS	WEIGHTS/MEASURES	YIELD ADJUST.	METHOD
Sliced peeled cucumbers . . . . .4 pounds, 8 ounces Salt . . . . .1½ tablespoons Finely chopped onions . . . . . . .2 cups Dehydrated parsley. . . . . .1/4 cup			1. Combine cucumbers, salt, onions and parsley; mix lightly; refrigerate for 2 hours.
Mayonnaise . . . . .2 cups			2. Add mayonnaise to cucumber mixture. Do not drain cucumbers and do not substitute salad dressing for mayonnaise; it will not give the same results. Mix lightly; refrigerate until used. Toss lightly again just before serving.

Potato Salad

Refer to footnotes for special dietary information

INGREDIENTS WEIGHTS/MEASURES	YIELD ADJUST.	METHOD
Red potatoes . . . . .12 pounds		1. Wash potatoes; cook in a steamer or stock pot. Drain potatoes well; cool to room temperature. 2. Peel potatoes; dice or slice them.
Finely chopped celery . . . . . . .3 cups Chopped hard-cooked eggs . . .12 Chopped drained pimiento. . . .1/2 cup Finely chopped onions . . . . . . .1 cup Salad mustard. . . . . .1/2 cup Salt .2 tablespoons Salad dressing . . . . .1 quart		3. Combine celery, eggs, pimiento, onions, mustard, salt and salad dressing in bottom of a large mixing bowl; mix well. 4. Add potatoes to salad dressing mixture; mix lightly until potatoes are well coated with dressing. 5. Chill thoroughly.

YIELD
50 portions (about 1 1/2 gallons)

PORTION SIZE
1/2 cup (No. 8 dipper)

NOTE
10 pounds pre-peeled potatoes may be used in step 1.

DIETARY INFORMATION
May be used as written for general, no added salt and bland diets. Diabetic diets — substitute cooked diabetic salad dressing for dressing in step 3. Each serving, using cooked diabetic salad dressing, provides 1 1/2 bread exchanges for 1/2 cup serving and 1 bread exchange for 1/3 cup serving.

YIELD
50 portions (about 2¹/₄ gallons)

PORTION SIZE
³/₄ cup

DIETARY INFORMATION
May be used as written for general, no added salt and low cholesterol diets. Diabetic diets — use diabetic French dressing in step 1. Each serving, using diabetic dressing, provides ¹/₂ bread exchange.

Frijole Salad

Refer to footnotes for special dietary information

INGREDIENTS	WEIGHTS/MEASURES	YIELD ADJUST.	METHOD
Drained and rinsed canned red kidney beans. . . . . .1¹/₂ quarts French dressing . . . . .1 quart			1. Combine beans and dressing; mix well and refrigerate 4 hours to overnight.
Shredded cabbage . . . . .1³/₄ gallons (about 4 pounds) Diced fresh tomatoes . . . . .2 quarts (about 2¹/₂ pounds) Chopped celery. . . . . .2 cups Chopped onions . . . . .2 cups			2. Place cabbage in large bowl; top with tomatoes, celery, onions and marinated beans; toss lightly and serve.

Hot Potato Salad

Refer to footnotes for special dietary information

INGREDIENTS	WEIGHTS/MEASURES	YIELD ADJUST.	METHOD
Chopped bacon . . . . .1 pound Chopped onions . . . . .1½ cups			1. Fry bacon until crisp; add onions; continue to cook over low heat until onions are soft but not brown.
Vinegar . . . . .1½ cups Water. . . . . .3 cups Salt . . . . .1 tablespoon Sugar. . . . . .¾ cup			2. Add vinegar, water, salt and sugar to bacon and onions. Mix well; heat to boiling point.
Sliced cooked potatoes . . . . . .10 pounds 8 ounces (1½ gallons) Chopped celery. . . . . .1 cup			3. Put potatoes and celery in a large mixing bowl. Pour hot dressing over them; mix lightly. Put salad in a shallow pan, cover and refrigerate 2 to 3 hours to allow flavor to develop. 4. Cover pan with aluminum foil, reheat in oven before serving. The length of time required will depend upon depth of the salad in the pan. Do not allow salad to cook in the oven.

YIELD
50 portions (about 1½ gallons)

PORTION SIZE
½ cup (No. 8 dipper)

TEMPERATURE
350°F. Oven

DIETARY INFORMATION
May be used as written for general and bland diets. Diabetic diets — omit sugar in step 2. Each serving, using sugar substitute, provides 1 bread and 1 fat exchange. Low cholesterol diets — omit bacon in step 1. Substitute ½ cup vegetable oil for the bacon fat.

YIELD
50 portions (about 1½ gallons)

PORTION SIZE
½ cup (No. 8 dipper)

VARIATION
Cottage cheese salad: Serve ¼ cup plain cottage cheese garnished with paprika on a lettuce leaf. Each portion will provide 1 ounce protein.

DIETARY INFORMATION
May be used as written for general and no added salt diets. Diabetic diets — each serving provides 1 lean meat exchange. Bland diets—omit green peppers in step 1. Low cholesterol diets — drain cottage cheese well before it is used or use cottage cheese with skim milk. Each serving provides the equivalent of 1 ounce of meat.

Garden Cottage Cheese

Refer to footnotes for special dietary information

INGREDIENTS	WEIGHTS/MEASURES	YIELD ADJUST.	METHOD

Chopped radishes . . . . .1½ cups
Finely chopped green onions . .1 cup
Finely chopped celery . . . . . . .1 quart
Finely chopped fresh green
  peppers . . . . .1½ cups
Finely diced peeled
  cucumbers . . . . .1 quart
			1. Combine radishes, green onions, celery, fresh green peppers and cucumbers; toss lightly.

Salt . . . . .1 tablespoon
Salad dressing . . . . .½ cup
Cottage cheese. . . . . .6 pounds,
  8 ounces
  (3½ quarts)
			2. Add salt to salad dressing; add to vegetables; mix lightly; add cottage cheese to vegetables; mix lightly but well. Refrigerate until served. (Prepare this salad as close to serving time as possible.)

Garden Vegetable Salad

Refer to footnotes for special dietary information

INGREDIENTS	WEIGHTS/MEASURES	YIELD ADJUST.	METHOD
Lettuce . . . . .2 pounds			1. Trim, wash and drain lettuce. Tear lettuce into bite-size pieces and put it in a large mixing bowl.
Shredded carrots . . . . .3 cups Chopped celery. . . . . .2 cups Chopped fresh green peppers .2 cups			2. Add carrots, celery and fresh green peppers to lettuce; toss together lightly; cover salad; refrigerate until served.
Tomato wedges (optional). . . . .50 wedges (7 or 8 tomatoes)			3. The salad may be garnished with tomato wedges, if desired, after it is put into salad bowls. 4. Do not add any salad dressing to vegetables until just before salad is served.

YIELD
50 portions (about 1½ gallons)

PORTION SIZE
½ cup

DIETARY INFORMATION
May be used as written for general, no added salt, bland and low cholesterol diets. Diabetic diets — each serving provides ½ vegetable exchange. Low fat and bland diets — omit fresh green peppers in step 2.

Sauerkraut Salad

Refer to footnotes for special dietary information

YIELD
50 portions (about 1½ gallons)

PORTION SIZE
½ cup

DIETARY INFORMATION

May be used as written for general, no added salt and low cholesterol diets. Diabetic diets — omit sugar. Use sugar substitute and syrup drained from fruit canned without sugar in step 2. Add sugar substitute to taste in step 2. Each serving using sugar substitute and juice from fruit canned without sugar provides 1 vegetable and 1 fat exchanges. Bland diets — omit fresh green peppers.

INGREDIENTS	WEIGHTS/MEASURES	YIELD ADJUST.	METHOD
Drained and chopped sauerkraut.............4½ quarts (1½ No. 10 cans) Thinly sliced celery..........3 cups Diced fresh green peppers....2 cups Grated carrots..............3 cups Finely chopped onions.......3 cups			1. Place sauerkraut, celery, green peppers, carrots and onions in mixing bowl; toss lightly. (If a milder salad is desired, rinse sauerkraut with clear water and drain well before it is combined with the other vegetables.)
Sugar...................1 quart Juice drained from peaches, pears or pineapple canned in heavy syrup...........3½ cups Vinegar..................2 cups Salad oil ....1½ cups			2. Combine sugar, fruit syrup, vinegar and oil together; add to sauerkraut mixture. Toss to coat all of the salad with dressing. Refrigerate at least 4 hours and preferably overnight. 3. Drain well and serve chilled.

Kidney Bean Salad

Refer to footnotes for special dietary information

INGREDIENTS	WEIGHTS/MEASURES	YIELD ADJUST.	METHOD
Canned kidney beans . . . . .3 quarts (1 No. 10 can)			1. Drain beans well; wash under running cold water; drain well.
Salad dressing . . . . .3 cups Salt .1½ tablespoons Vinegar . . . . .½ cup			2. Combine dressing, salt and vinegar in a large mixing bowl; mix well; add beans; stir lightly to coat beans well with dressing.
Chopped hard-cooked eggs . . .24 Chopped celery. . . . . .1 quart Finely chopped onions. . . . . . .1 cup Chopped fresh green peppers .1 cup Sweet pickle relish . . . . .2 cups Diced American process or cheddar cheese . . . . .1 pound, 8 ounces			3. Add eggs, celery, onions, green peppers, pickle and cheese to beans; mix well. 4. Cover and refrigerate until served.

YIELD
50 portions (about 1½ gallons)

PORTION SIZE
½ cup (No. 8 dipper)

DIETARY INFORMATION
May be used as written for general diets. Diabetic diets — substitute cooked diabetic salad dressing for dressing in step 2. Each serving, using cooked diabetic salad dressing, provides 1½ bread and 1 high fat meat exchanges for ½ cup serving and 1 bread and 1 lean meat exchanges for ⅓ cup serving. No added salt diets — omit pickle relish. Bland diets — omit fresh green peppers. Each serving provides the equivalent of 1 ounce meat.

203

YIELD
50 portions (about 1½ gallons)

PORTION SIZE
½ cup (No. 8 dipper)

NOTE
Equal amounts of other types of beans may be substituted for the beans in the basic recipe.

DIETARY INFORMATION
May be used as written for general, no added salt and low cholesterol diets. Diabetic diets — substitute cooked diabetic salad dressing for dressing in step 1. Each serving, using cooked diabetic salad dressing, provides 2 vegetable exchanges.

Three-Bean Salad

Refer to footnotes for special dietary information

INGREDIENTS	WEIGHTS/MEASURES	YIELD ADJUST.	METHOD
Canned drained green beans . .2 quarts Canned drained wax beans . . .2 quarts Canned drained lima beans . . .2 quarts Italian-style salad dressing. . . .2 cups			1. Put drained beans in a large mixing bowl; pour salad dressing over beans; mix well; cover and refrigerate 1 to 2 hours for beans to absorb flavor of salad dressing.
Finely chopped onions . . . . . . .1½ cups Finely chopped celery . . . . . . .1½ cups Chopped fresh green peppers .1 cup			2. Add onions, celery and green peppers to beans; chill thoroughly. 3. Add a little more salad dressing, if necessary, just before salad is served.

Sliced Tomato Salad

Refer to footnotes for special dietary information

INGREDIENTS	WEIGHTS/MEASURES	YIELD ADJUST.	METHOD
Fresh tomatoes. . . . . .10 pounds			1. Wash tomatoes. Remove top portion of the tomato core and cut each tomato into about ¼-inch thick slices.
Lettuce . . . . .2 to 3 heads			2. Trim, wash and drain lettuce. Separate lettuce into leaves; arrange a lettuce leaf on each plate or on sheet pans. 3. Arrange 2 to 4 tomato slices on each lettuce leaf, just before salad is served. 4. Do not add any salad dressing, if it is used, until just before salad is served.

YIELD
50 portions

PORTION SIZE
2 to 4 slices tomato

DIETARY INFORMATION
May be used as written for general, no added salt, bland, low fat and low cholesterol diets. Diabetic diets — each serving provides 1 vegetable exchange.

YIELD
50 portions

PORTION SIZE
2 to 3 tomato slices
1/4 cup cottage cheese

DIETARY INFORMATION
May be used as written for general, no added salt, bland and low fat diets. Diabetic diets — each serving provides 1 vegetable and 1 lean meat exchanges. Low cholesterol diets — drain any cream from cottage cheese before it is used in step 4. Each serving provides the equivalent of 1 ounce cooked meat.

Tomato and Cottage Cheese Salad

Refer to footnotes for special dietary information

INGREDIENTS	WEIGHTS/MEASURES	YIELD ADJUST.	METHOD
Fresh tomatoes	7 pounds		1. Wash tomatoes; remove top portion of the tomato core; cut tomatoes into slices about 1/4 inch thick.
Lettuce	2 to 3 heads		2. Trim, wash and drain lettuce. Separate lettuce into leaves; arrange a lettuce leaf on each salad plate or on sheet pans.
Cottage cheese	6 pounds, 8 ounces (3 1/2 quarts)		3. Arrange 2 or 3 tomato slices according to size of slices, on each lettuce cup. 4. Put a level No. 16 scoop (1/4 cup) cottage cheese in the center of the tomato slices. 5. Do not add any salad dressing until just before salad is served.

Tossed Salad Combinations

Refer to footnotes for special dietary information

INGREDIENTS	WEIGHTS/MEASURES	YIELD ADJUST.	METHOD
No. I			1. Cut or chop lettuce into bite-size pieces. Clean and chop or shred other vegetables; toss lightly and refrigerate until used.
Lettuce . . . . .2 large heads			
Chopped green onions . . . . . . .1 quart			2. Do not add diced tomatoes until ready to serve salad.
Fresh diced tomatoes. . . . . . .2 quarts			
Diced or sliced peeled			
cucumbers . . . . .2 quarts			
No. II			
Lettuce . . . . .2 large heads			
Escarole . . . . .1 head			
Romaine . . . . .1 head			
Endive. . . . . .1 head			
No. III			
Lettuce . . . . .2 large heads			
Shredded cabbage . . . . .1 quart			
Chopped celery. . . . . .2 quarts			
Diced or sliced peeled			
cucumbers . . . . .1 quart			
Fresh diced tomatoes. . . . . . .2 quarts			

YIELD
50 portions (about 2¼ gallons)

PORTION SIZE
¾ cup

DIETARY INFORMATION
May be used as written for general, no added salt and bland diets. Diabetic diets — each serving provides ½ vegetable exchange.

Cooked Salad Dressing for Diabetics

Refer to footnotes for special dietary information

YIELD
1 quart

PORTION SIZE
1 tablespoon

PAN SIZE
2-quart double boiler

DIETARY INFORMATION
May be used as written for general, no added salt, bland, soft and mechanical soft diets. Diabetic diets — up to 2 tablespoons may be considered free. Low cholesterol diets — omit eggs. Use 1 cup liquid egg substitute in step 1.

INGREDIENTS	WEIGHTS/MEASURES	YIELD ADJUST.	METHOD
Slightly beaten eggs	1 cup (5 to 6 medium)		1. Combine all ingredients in the top of a double boiler; cook and stir over boiling water until thickened. Remove from heat and refrigerate until used.
Cold water.	3 cups		
Cornstarch	¼ cup		
Dry mustard	1 tablespoon		
Vinegar	3 tablespoons		
Celery seed (optional).	2 teaspoons		
Salt	1 teaspoon		

French Dressing for Diabetics

Refer to footnotes for special dietary information

INGREDIENTS	WEIGHTS/MEASURES	YIELD ADJUST.	METHOD
Dry mustard . . . . .1 tablespoon Paprika . . . . .2 teaspoons Chopped onions . . . . .¼ cup Vinegar . . . . .¼ cup Vegetable oil . . . . .2 tablespoons Crushed canned tomatoes with juice. . . . . .2 cups Water. .1⅓ cups Cornstarch . . . . .2 teaspoons			1. Combine mustard, paprika, onions, vinegar, oil, tomatoes, water and cornstarch in a blender or food processor and blend on high speed until smooth; pour into saucepan and cook and stir over medium heat until slightly thickened. Remove from heat and cool to room temperature.

Sugar substitute . . . . .Equal to 3
                    tablespoons
                    sugar
			2. Add to dressing; stir to mix and serve at room temperature.

YIELD
1 quart

PORTION SIZE
1 tablespoon

PAN SIZE
2-quart saucepan

DIETARY INFORMATION
May be used as written for general, no added salt, low cholesterol and mechanical soft diets. Diabetic diets — up to 2 tablespoons may be considered free.

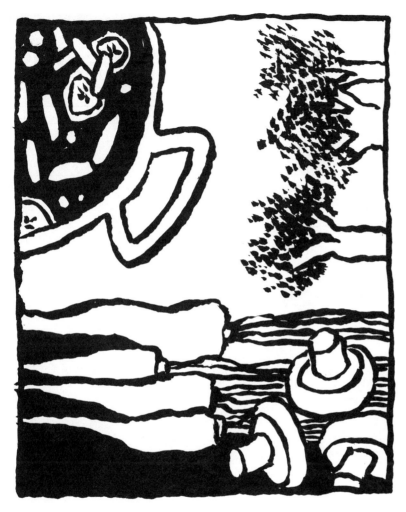

Chapter 10
Vegetables

Information   **212**

Vegetable Information

PROPER CARE AND USE OF VEGETABLES

1. Vegetables should always be prepared as close to serving time as possible.
2. Vegetables should never be overcooked.
3. Baking soda should not be used in cooking vegetables because it destroys vitamins in the vegetables.
4. Vegetable juices, except for cabbage and some other strong vegetables, should be saved and used in gravies and soups. The use of vegetable juices will improve both the flavor and the nutritive value of gravies and soups.
5. Vegetables should not be soaked in water a long time before or after cooking. Long soaking will remove some of the vitamins in the vegetables.
6. Vegetables should be started to cook in boiling water. Vegetables should not be put in cold water and brought to a boil unless the recipe includes such specific instructions.
7. Vegetables should be handled carefully before and after cooking to prevent breaking and give them a more attractive appearance.
8. Cooking times for vegetables should be followed carefully in each recipe.
9. Vegetables should be cut into uniform, manageable-size pieces; they should not be too large to handle nor should they be chopped or pureed except for special diets.
10. Vegetables should generally be cooked in as small an amount of water as possible, except for a few strong vegetables where the recipe instructions include the use of more water.

Guidelines for Cooking Frozen Vegetables

YIELD 50 portions (about 1 1/2 gallons) **EACH PORTION** 1/2 cup to (3 to 4 ounces)

KIND OF VEGETABLE	AMOUNT TO BUY	APPROX. AMOUNT OF WATER TO USE	APPROX. TIME TO COOK	METHOD
Asparagus	10 pounds	3 1/2 quarts	8 to 10 minutes	1. Tap frozen vegetables in package lightly to break up blocks
Green or wax beans	10 pounds	1 gallon	10 to 15 minutes	2. Bring water to a boil in a stock pot or steam-jacketed kettle.
French-style green beans	10 pounds	3 quarts	6 to 8 minutes	3. Add 1 teaspoon salt for each quart of water.
Lima beans	10 pounds	1 gallon	12 to 14 minutes	4. Add vegetables; bring the water back to a boil.
Broccoli	10 pounds	1 gallon	7 to 9 minutes	5. Reduce heat and cook, uncovered, until vegetables are just tender. Lima beans, cauliflower,
Brussels sprouts	10 pounds	3 1/2 quarts	7 to 10 minutes	corn, succotash and summer squash are cooked covered.
Cauliflower	10 pounds	1 1/2 gallons	4 to 6 minutes	6. Drain vegetables; save liquid for use in soups, sauces and gravies. Add margarine, if desired,
Whole kernel corn	10 pounds	1 gallon	6 to 10 minutes	and serve hot.
Mustard or turnip greens	10 pounds	1 gallon	15 to 35 minutes	
Mixed vegetables	10 pounds	1 gallon	10 to 14 minutes	
Okra	10 pounds	1 gallon	5 to 8 minutes	
Peas or peas and carrots	10 pounds	3 quarts	8 to 10 minutes	
Spinach	10 pounds	1 quart	5 to 10 minutes	
Summer squash	10 pounds	1 quart	10 minutes	
Succotash	10 pounds	1 gallon	12 to 14 minutes	

Guidelines for Using Canned Vegetables

1. Food should not be used from any can which bulges, leaks, is dented at the seams or has liquid which is milky, off-color or foamy.

2. Canned vegetables should be simmered in their own juice 10 to 12 minutes except for beets and spinach which should be simmered 20 minutes, in order to kill any harmful bacteria which might be in the canned foods.

3. Generally speaking, one No. 10 can of canned vegetables will yield about 24 1/2-cup portions.

4. Canned vegetables should be heated as closely as possible to serving time.

5. After canned vegetables are heated, they should be drained and put into serving pans. Add 1/2 cup (1 stick) margarine for each No. 10 can of vegetables used.

6. Leftover vegetables should be covered and refrigerated as soon as possible.

Guidelines for Steaming Vegetables

YIELD 50 portions (about 1 1/2 gallons)

EACH PORTION 1/2 cup to (3 to 4 ounces)

KIND OF VEGETABLE	WEIGHT	APPROX. TIME TO STEAM AT 5 POUNDS PRESSURE	METHOD
Frozen green beans	10 pounds	15 to 18 minutes	1. Put frozen vegetables in a steamer pan. Cover winter squash with a lid or aluminum foil.
Frozen lima beans	10 pounds	12 to 15 minutes	2. Begin counting time when the gauge registers 5 pounds pressure.
Frozen broccoli	10 pounds	8 to 10 minutes	3. Cook vegetables the length of time on chart. Test vegetables to see if they are done; drain well. Teh length of time for steaming vegetables will vary with the tenderness of the vegetables.
Frozen Brussels sprouts	10 pounds	8 to 10 minutes	
Fresh carrots (as purchased)	13 pounds	10 to 12 minutes	
Frozen cauliflower	10 pounds	8 to 10 minutes	
Frozen whole kernel corn	10 pounds	8 to 10 minutes	4. Add 1/2 cup (1 stick) melted margarine and 2 teaspoons salt for each 5 pounds of cooked vegetables.
Frozen peas	10 pounds	8 to 10 minutes	
Fresh white potatoes, whole*		20 to 25 minutes	
Fresh white potatoes, quartered*		18 to 22 minutes	
Fresh white potatoes, diced*		10 to 12 minutes	
Mixed vegetables	10 pounds	12 to 15 minutes	
Frozen spinach (partially thawed)	10 pounds	8 to 10 minutes	
Frozen winter squash partially thawed)	10 pounds	8.to 10 minutes	

*The amount of potatoes necessary to serve 50 portions will vary with the recipe used but will be from about 12 pounds 8 ounces to 15 pounds, as purchased.

NOTES 1. VEGETABLES SHOULD BE COOKED IN SMALL BATCHES.

2. Vegetables should be cooked as near to serving time as possible.

3. Any leftover vegetables should be covered and refrigerated as soon as possible.

Guidelines for Cooking Fresh Vegetables

YIELD 25 portions (about 3 quarts)

EACH PORTION 1/2 cup to (3 to 4 ounces)

KIND OF VEGETABLE	AMOUNT TO BUY	APPROX. AMOUNT OF WATER TO USE	APPROX. TIME TO COOK	METHOD
Asparagus	9 pounds	1 1/2 quarts	10 to 20 minutes	1. Bring the water to a boil in a heavy stock pot or steam-jacketed kettle.
Green or wax beans	6 pounds	2 quarts	20 to 30 minutes	2. Add 1 teaspoon salt for each quart of water.
Beets	7 pounds	to cover	60 to 90 minutes	3. Add vegetables and bring water back to a boil. Cook until vegetables are just tender.
Broccoli	7 pounds	3 quarts	10 to 12 minutes	4. Drain vegetables; save juice for use in soups, sauces and gravies. Add margarine, if desired, and
Brussels sprouts	7 pounds	3 quarts	10 to 15 minutes	serve hot.
Cabbage	6 pounds, 8 ounces	3 quarts	10 to 12 minutes	
Carrots	6 pounds, 8 ounces	2 quarts	15 to 20 minutes	
Cauliflower	12 pounds, 8 ounces	3 quarts	12 minutes	
Corn on the cob	12 pounds, 12 ounces	to cover	16 minutes	
Eggplant	5 pounds	to cover	5 to 10 minutes	
Greens	7 pounds	1 quart	20 to 30 minutes	
Onions	5 pounds, 8 ounces	3 quarts	15 to 20 minutes	
Parsnips	6 pounds	to cover	20 minutes	
Sweet potatoes	8 pounds	to cover	25 to 35 minutes	
White potatoes	8 pounds	to cover	20 to 25 minutes	
Summer squash	6 pounds	1 cup	20 minutes	
Turnips	6 pounds	2 quarts	20 to 30 minutes	

NOTES 1. Peel and prepare vegetables as close to serving time as possible.

2. Cooking times for fresh vegetables will vary according to the age and tenderness of the vegetables.

3. Cook vegetables in small quantities and as near to serving time as possible.

4. Any leftover vegetables should be covered and refrigerated as soon as possible.

YIELD
50 portions (about 1½ gallons)

PORTION SIZE
½ cup (No. 8 dipper)

PAN SIZE
Heavy 3-gallon stock pot
Roasting pan

TEMPERATURE
350°F. Oven

VARIATION
Italian-style baked beans: Fry 1 quart chopped celery and 3 minced garlic cloves with onions in step 1. Add 1 teaspoon basil and 2 teaspoons oregano with seasonings in step 2.

DIETARY INFORMATION
May be used as written for general diets.

Baked Beans

Refer to footnotes for special dietary information

INGREDIENTS	WEIGHTS/MEASURES	YIELD ADJUST.	METHOD
Chopped bacon . . . . .1 pound Chopped onions . . . . .2 cups			1. Fry bacon in a heavy pot until crisp; add onions to bacon; continue to cook until onions are golden. Do not drain fat from bacon and onions.
Canned pork and beans . . . . . .1½ gallons (2 No. 10 cans) Brown sugar . . . . .2 cups Salad mustard. . . . . .¼ cup Catsup . . . . .1 cup			2. Add beans, sugar, mustard and catsup to onions and bacon; mix well. 3. Pour beans into roasting pan; bake, uncovered, 1½ hours or until browned.

Creole Green Beans

Refer to footnotes for special dietary information

INGREDIENTS	WEIGHTS/MEASURES	YIELD ADJUST.	METHOD
Bacon fat . . . . .1/2 cup Chopped onions . . . . .2 cups Chopped fresh green peppers .1 cup			1. Fry onions and peppers in bacon fat until onions are golden.
All-purpose flour . . . . .1/2 cup Tomato juice . . . . .2 quarts			2. Stir flour into fat and vegetable mixture; cook and stir until smooth. Add tomato juice to flour mixture; cook and stir 5 to 10 minutes or until smooth.
Canned green beans. . . . . . . .1 1/2 gallons (2 No. 10 cans) Salt . . . . .1 tablespoon Pepper. . . . . .1/2 teaspoon			3. Simmer green beans in their own liquid 10 to 12 minutes; drain well; add to tomato sauce along with salt and pepper. Serve hot.

YIELD
50 portions (about 1 1/2 gallons)

PORTION SIZE
1/2 cup (4 ounces)

PAN SIZE
Heavy 3-gallon stock pot

VARIATION
Creole wax beans: Use 2 No. 10 cans of yellow wax beans instead of green beans in step 3.

NOTE
10 pounds frozen green beans may be cooked 15 minutes in 1 gallon salted boiling water, drained and used instead of canned beans in step 3. It is not necessary to simmer frozen beans for the additional 12 minutes.

DIETARY INFORMATION
May be used as written for general diets. Diabetic diets — each serving provides 1 vegetable exchange. Bland diets — omit pepper and fresh green peppers. Low cholesterol diets — omit bacon fat. Fry vegetables in vegetable oil in step 1.

YIELD
50 portions (about 1½ gallons)

PORTION SIZE
½ cup (4 ounces)

PAN SIZE
Heavy 3-gallon stock pot

VARIATIONS
1. Southern-style green beans: Cook 1 pound chopped bacon until fat is transparent; add partially cooked bacon to beans and cook the bacon with the beans in step 1. Use bacon fat to fry onions in step 2.
2. Lyonnaise wax beans: Use 2 No. 10 cans of yellow wax beans instead of green beans in step 1.

NOTE
8 pounds, 8 ounces frozen green beans may be cooked 15 minutes in 1 gallon salted boiling water, drained and used instead of the canned green beans in step 1. It is not necessary to simmer frozen beans the additional 10 to 12 minutes.

DIETARY INFORMATION
May be used as written for general, no added salt and low cholesterol diets. Diabetic diets — each serving provides 1 vegetable exchange. Bland diets — omit pepper.

Lyonnaise Green Beans

Refer to footnotes for special dietary information

INGREDIENTS	WEIGHTS/MEASURES	YIELD ADJUST.	METHOD
Canned green beans	1½ gallons (2 No. 10 cans)		1. Simmer beans in their own liquid 10 to 12 minutes; drain beans well; return to pot.
Chopped onions	2 quarts		2. Fry onions in margarine until light yellow.
Margarine	½ cup (4 ounces)		3. Add onions and fat with salt and pepper to hot beans; mix well; serve hot.
Salt	1½ tablespoons		
Pepper	½ teaspoon		

Harvard Beets

Refer to footnotes for special dietary information

INGREDIENTS	WEIGHTS/MEASURES	YIELD ADJUST.	METHOD
Canned beets	1½ gallons (2 No. 10 cans)		1. Simmer beets in their own liquid 20 minutes; drain beets well; keep 1 quart beet juice for use in step 2.
Cornstarch	½ cup		2. Combine cornstarch and water; mix until smooth; add to hot beet juice; add cloves, cinnamon, sugar and salt; cook and stir 5 minutes over moderate heat or until smooth and thickened. Remove sauce from heat.
Cold water	2 cups		
Beet juice	1 quart		
Ground cloves	½ teaspoon		
Ground cinnamon	1 teaspoon		
Sugar	1 cup		
Salt	1 teaspoon		
Margarine	½ cup (4 ounces)		3. Add margarine and vinegar to hot sauce; stir until well blended.
Vinegar	¾ cup		4. Pour sauce over hot beets and serve hot.

YIELD
50 portions (about 1½ gallons)

PORTION SIZE
½ cup (4 ounces)

PAN SIZE
Heavy 3-gallon stock pot

DIETARY INFORMATION
May be used as written for general, no added salt, low fat, low cholesterol and soft diets. Diabetic diets — omit sugar. Add sugar substitute to taste at the end of step 2. Each serving, using sugar substitute, provides 1 vegetable exchange. Bland diets — omit cloves.

YIELD
50 portions (about 1½ gallons)

PORTION SIZE
½ cup (4 ounces)

PAN SIZE
Heavy 3-gallon stock pot

DIETARY INFORMATION
May be used as written for general, no added salt, bland, low fat, low cholesterol and soft diets. Diabetic diets — omit sugar. Sweeten to taste with sugar substitute at the end of step 3. Each serving with sugar substitute provides ½ bread exchange.

Orange-Glazed Beets

Refer to footnotes for special dietary information

INGREDIENTS	WEIGHTS/MEASURES	YIELD ADJUST.	METHOD
Sliced canned beets	1½ gallons (2 No. 10 cans)		1. Simmer beets in their own liquid 20 minutes; drain beets well; keep 1½ quarts beet juice for use in step 2.
Cornstarch . . . . Salt . . . . Sugar. Cold water. . . . . Beet juice	¾ cup 1 tablespoon 1½ cups 2 cups 1½ quarts		2. Combine cornstarch, salt, sugar and water; mix until smooth; add to hot beet juice; cook and stir over moderate heat 5 minutes or until smooth and clear.
Margarine . . . . Orange juice . . . . Lemon juice	½ cup (4 ounces) 1 cup 1 cup		3. Add margarine, orange and lemon juice to hot sauce; stir until well blended. 4. Pour sauce over hot beets; serve hot.

Brussels Sprouts with Cheese Sauce

Refer to footnotes for special dietary information

INGREDIENTS	WEIGHTS/MEASURES	YIELD ADJUST.	METHOD
Frozen Brussels sprouts......10 pounds Salt......................1 tablespoon Boiling water...............1 gallon			1. Tap package of Brussels sprouts lightly to break up solid blocks; add to boiling salted water; return to a boil; cook 7 to 10 minutes or until tender but not soggy. Drain and set aside for use in step 4.
All-purpose flour............1½ cups Nonfat dry milk.............2 cups Salt......................1½ teaspoons Margarine, melted..........1 cup (8 ounces)			2. Sift flour, dry milk and salt together; add to margarine in a heavy pot; cook and stir over low heat until smooth but do not let brown.
Cold water................3 quarts			3. Add cold water to flour mixture; cook and stir over medium heat until sauce is smooth and thickened and the starchy taste is gone.
Shredded or ground American process cheese..........1 pound, 8 ounces Grated Parmesan cheese.....½ cup Salad mustard.............2 tablespoons			4. Add cheese and mustard to sauce; stir until smooth over low heat; pour over hot Brussels sprouts.

YIELD
50 portions (about 1½ gallons)

PORTION SIZE
½ cup (4 ounces)

PAN SIZE
Heavy 3-gallon stock pot

VARIATIONS
1. Green beans with cheese sauce: Simmer 2 No. 10 cans green beans in their own juice 10 to 12 minutes; drain well; serve with hot cheese sauce made as directed in basic recipe.
2. Cabbage with cheese sauce: Clean and shred 11 pounds of cabbage. Drop cabbage into 2 quarts boiling salted water; cover tightly; bring to a boil. Cook for 12 minutes, drain well; stir into hot cheese sauce made as directed in basic recipe. (It is important not to increase the amount of cooking water and to cover pot tightly because the cabbage should cook in the steam in the pot.)
3. Cauliflower with cheese sauce: Cook cauliflower 10 to 12 minutes in salted boiling water; drain well and serve with hot cheese sauce made as directed by the basic recipe.

DIETARY INFORMATION
May be used as written for general, no added salt, bland and low cholesterol diets. Diabetic diets — each serving provides 1 vegetable, ½ lowfat milk and 2 fat exchanges.

YIELD
50 portions

PORTION SIZE
1 wedge

DIETARY INFORMATION
May be used as written for general diets. Diabetic diets — each serving provides 1 vegetable exchange. No added salt diets — cook wedges in salt-free broth or plain water.

Cabbage Wedges

Refer to footnotes for special dietary information

INGREDIENTS WEIGHTS/MEASURES	YIELD ADJUST.	METHOD

Fresh cabbage . . . . .12 pounds
Boiling ham or corned beef
   stock with most of the fat
   removed . . . . .as necessary
		1. Trim and wash cabbage; cut into 50 wedges. Do not remove cores. Put wedges in a roasting pan; cover with hot stock. (Prepare stock using ham soup and gravy base if fresh stock is not available.)
		2. Return roaster to heat; simmer uncovered 10 to 12 minutes or until tender. Do not overcook.

Salt . . . . .as necessary		3. Remove cabbage from stock with a slotted spoon or skimmer to a steam table pan. Add salt, if necessary; serve hot.

Shredded Cabbage

Refer to footnotes for special dietary information

INGREDIENTS	WEIGHTS/MEASURES	YIELD ADJUST.	METHOD
Fresh cabbage . . . . .11 pounds Salt .1½ tablespoons Boiling water. . . . . .2 quarts			1. Trim and wash cabbage. Shred coarsely; add to boiling salted water; cover tightly; cook cabbage in steam for 12 minutes; drain well.
Margarine, melted. . . . . .½ cup (4 ounces) Pepper. . . . . .1 teaspoon			2. Pour melted butter or margarine over cabbage; sprinkle pepper over cabbage; mix lightly to coat cabbage with butter or margarine and pepper. Serve hot.

YIELD
50 portions (about 1½ gallons)

PORTION SIZE
½ cup (3 to 4 ounces)

PAN SIZE
Heavy 5-gallon stock pot

VARIATION
Country style cabbage: Omit butter or margarine in step 2. Fry 1 pound chopped bacon until crisp in a heavy pot. (Do not drain fat from bacon.) Add cooked cabbage and pepper to bacon and toss lightly. Serve hot.

DIETARY INFORMATION
May be used as written for general, no added salt and low cholesterol diets. Diabetic diets — each serving provides 1 vegetable exchange. Bland diets — omit pepper.

YIELD
50 portions (1 pan)

PORTION SIZE
½ cup

PAN SIZE
12 × 20 × 4-inch steam table pan

TEMPERATURE
350°F. Oven

DIETARY INFORMATION
May be used as written for general diets. Diabetic diets — each serving provides 1 bread, 1 vegetable and 1 fat exchanges. Low cholesterol diets — omit eggs. Use 2 cups liquid egg substitute or 2 cups egg whites in step 3.

Escalloped Corn and Broccoli

Refer to footnotes for special dietary information

INGREDIENTS	WEIGHTS/MEASURES	YIELD ADJUST.	METHOD
Frozen chopped broccoli . . . . . 5 pounds			1. Cook broccoli according to directions on the package until barely tender.
Finely chopped onions . . . . 1½ quarts Margarine . . . . 1 cup (8 ounces)			2. Fry onions in heavy frying pan over medium heat, using as much margarine as necessary, until onions are soft but not browned. Add remaining margarine and heat only to melt the margarine. Remove from heat and cool to lukewarm.
Cream-style canned corn . . . . . 3 quarts (1 No. 10 can) Slightly beaten eggs . . . . 2 cups (10-12 medium) Salt . . . . 1 tablespoon Pepper . . . . ½ teaspoon Dry bread crumbs . . . . 3 cups (12 ounces) Skim milk . . . . 1 cup			3. Mix corn, eggs, salt, pepper, bread crumbs and milk together to blend. Add onions and margarine and mix lightly; add broccoli and mix lightly. Pour mixture into well-greased pan. 4. Bake 45 minutes to 1 hour or until set and slightly puffy. Serve hot.

Corn Pudding

Refer to footnotes for special dietary information

INGREDIENTS	WEIGHTS/MEASURES	YIELD ADJUST.	METHOD
Cream-style corn . . . . .1½ gallons (2 No. 10 cans)			1. Combine all ingredients; heat to just below boiling, stirring constantly, over low heat.
Sugar .¼ cup			2. Pour corn mixture into a buttered baking pan; bake about 1 hour or until center is set. The pan may be placed in a pan of hot water to reduce danger of curdling.
Salt .2 tablespoons			
Milk .2 quarts			
Lightly beaten eggs . . . . .2 cups (10-12 medium)			
Soft bread crumbs . . . . .1 quart (12-13 ounces)			

YIELD
50 portions (about 1½ gallons)

PORTION SIZE
½ cup (4 ounces)

PAN SIZE
Roasting pan

TEMPERATURE
300°F. Oven

DIETARY INFORMATION
May be used as written for general, no added salt and bland diets. Diabetic diets — each ½ cup serving provides 1½ bread exchanges. Each ⅓ cup serving provides 1 bread exchange. Low cholesterol diets — omit eggs. Use 2 cups liquid egg substitute in step 1.

YIELD
50 portions (about 2¼ gallons)

PORTION SIZE
¾ cup (6 ounces)

PAN SIZE
Heavy 3-gallon stock pot
Roasting pan

TEMPERATURE
325°F. Oven

DIETARY INFORMATION
May be used as written for general and low cholesterol diets. Diabetic diets — each serving provides 2 bread and 1 fat exchanges. Bland diets — omit pepper.

Corn and Spaghetti

Refer to footnotes for special dietary information

INGREDIENTS	WEIGHTS/MEASURES	YIELD ADJUST.	METHOD
Spaghetti broken into about 2-inch pieces . . . . .2 pounds Salt . . . . .1 tablespoon Boiling water. . . . . .1½ gallons Vegetable oil . . . . .1 tablespoon			1. Stir spaghetti into boiling, salted water; add vegetable oil; cook 15 minutes or until tender; drain well; set aside for use in step 3.
Chopped bacon . . . . .2 pounds Chopped onions . . . . .3 cups			2. Fry bacon until crisp; drain well. Put ¼ cup bacon fat back in frying pan; fry onions in bacon fat until golden.
Cream-style corn. . . . . .4½ quarts (1½ No. 10 cans) Salt . . . . .1½ tablespoons Pepper. . . . . .½ teaspoon Paprika . . . . .1 teaspoon			3. Combine cooked spaghetti, onions, corn, drained bacon, salt, and pepper; mix lightly. 4. Pour corn mixture into well-greased roasting pan; sprinkle with paprika; bake 30 minutes.

Mexican Corn

Refer to footnotes for special dietary information

INGREDIENTS	WEIGHTS/MEASURES	YIELD ADJUST.	METHOD
Chopped fresh green peppers .3 cups Margarine . . . . .½ cup (4 ounces)			1. Fry green peppers in margarine in heavy pot until limp.
Canned whole-kernel corn . . . .1½ gallons (2 No. 10 cans)			2. Simmer corn in its own juice 10 to 12 minutes; drain well; add to peppers.
Salt . . . . .1½ tablespoons Sugar. . . . . .2 tablespoons Finely chopped pimiento . . . . .½ cup			3. Add salt, sugar and pimiento to hot corn and peppers; mix well and serve hot.

YIELD
50 portions (about 1½ gallons)

PORTION SIZE
½ cup (4 ounces)

PAN SIZE
Heavy 3-gallon stock pot

VARIATION
Corn O'Brien: Use 2 cups of chopped onions and 2 cups of chopped fresh green peppers instead of 3 cups of chopped fresh green peppers in step 1.

NOTE
10 pounds frozen whole-kernel corn may be cooked 10 minutes in 1 gallon salted boiling water and used instead of the canned corn in step 2.

DIETARY INFORMATION
May be used as written for general, no added salt and low cholesterol diets. diabetic diets — each serving provides 1 bread exchange. Bland diets — omit fresh green peppers.

YIELD
50 portions

PORTION SIZE
2 to 3 slices

PAN SIZE
18 × 26-inch sheet pans

TEMPERATURE
450°F. Oven

DIETARY INFORMATION
May be used as written for general, no added salt, bland and soft diets. Diabetic diets — each serving provides 1 bread and 1 fat exchanges. Low cholesterol diets — omit eggs. Use 2 cups liquid egg substitute in step 3. Use skim milk in step 3.

Oven-Browned Eggplant

Refer to footnotes for special dietary information

INGREDIENTS	WEIGHTS/MEASURES	YIELD ADJUST.	METHOD
Fresh eggplant	10 pounds (about 8 eggplants)		1. Peel eggplant and cut into slices about 1/3 to 1/2-inch thick.
All-purpose flour Salt	3 cups 1 1/2 tablespoons		2. Mix flour and salt together; dredge eggplant slices in seasoned flour.
Eggs Milk	2 cups (5-6 medium) 2 cups		3. Mix eggs and milk together until smooth. 4. Dip floured eggplant slices in egg mixture; drain slightly.
Dry bread crumbs Grated Parmesan cheese Salt Paprika Margarine, melted	1 1/4 quarts (1 pound, 4 ounces) 1 cup 2 tablespoons 1 tablespoon 1 1/2 cups (12 ounces)		5. Mix crumbs, cheese, salt and paprika together; dredge eggplant slices in crumb mixture and put on heavily buttered sheet pans being careful they do not touch each other. (The flour mixture, egg mixture and crumb mixture should be prepared ahead of time so you can work rapidly dipping slices first in flour mixture, then in the egg mixture, then in crumb mixture and onto sheet pan as smoothly as possible.) 6. Dribble melted margarine over slices of eggplant, being sure that each slice has some melted margarine. 7. Bake 15 minutes; turn slices over and bake another 10 minutes or until tender and browned.

Creamed Spinach

Refer to footnotes for special dietary information

INGREDIENTS	WEIGHTS/MEASURES	YIELD ADJUST.	METHOD
Frozen spinach . . . . .10 pounds Salt . . . . .1 tablespoon Boiling water. . . . . .2 quarts			1. (Spinach should be almost completely thawed.) Add spinach to boiling salted water; cook 8 minutes; drain well; chop spinach coarsely; reserve for use in step 4.
All-purpose flour . . . . .1½ cups Nonfat dry milk . . . . .2 cups Salt . . . . .1½ tablespoons Ground nutmeg. . . . . .2 teaspoons Margarine, melted. . . . . .½ cup (4 ounces)			2. Sift flour, milk, salt and nutmeg together; add to melted margarine in heavy pot; cook and stir over low heat until smooth, but not browned.
Cold water. . . . . .3 quarts			3. Add cold water to flour mixture; cook and stir over moderate heat until smooth and thickened and the starchy taste is gone. 4. Add chopped spinach to hot sauce; reheat over low heat. Serve hot. Do not stir creamed spinach any more than absolutely necessary. It is best to have spinach hot when sauce is finished, if possible.

YIELD
50 portions (about 1½ gallons)

PORTION SIZE
½ cup (No. 8 dipper)

PAN SIZE
Heavy 3-gallon pot

VARIATION
Creamed spinach with peanuts: Omit nutmeg in step 2. Add 2 cups finely chopped peanuts in step 4.

DIETARY INFORMATION
May be used as written for general, no added salt, low cholesterol, low fat and soft diets. Diabetic diets — each serving provides ½ bread exchange. For bland diet delete nutmeg.

YIELD
50 portions (about 1½ gallons)

PORTION SIZE
½ cup (3 to 4 ounces)

PAN SIZE
Heavy 3-gallon stock pot

DIETARY INFORMATION
May be used as written for general diets. Diabetic diets — each serving provides 1 vegetable and 1 fat exchanges. Bland diets — omit pepper.

Southern-Style Greens

Refer to footnotes for special dietary information

INGREDIENTS	WEIGHTS/MEASURES	YIELD ADJUST.	METHOD
Frozen mustard or turnip greens . . . . 10 pounds Salt . . . . 1½ tablespoons Boiling water . . . . 1 gallon Chopped bacon . . . . 1 pound			1. (Greens should be almost completely thawed.) Put greens in pot with salt, water and bacon; bring to a boil; cook gently, uncovered, 30 minutes or until tender. Drain well.
Pepper . . . . ½ teaspoon			2. Cut through greens several times with a sharp knife; sprinkle with pepper and serve hot.

Peas and Carrots

Refer to footnotes for special dietary information

INGREDIENTS	WEIGHTS/MEASURES	YIELD ADJUST.	METHOD
Frozen peas . . . . .5 pounds Boiling water. . . . . .2 quarts Salt . . . . .2 teaspoons			1. Add peas to boiling salted water; cook gently 15 to 20 minutes or until peas are tender. Drain well.
Diced fresh carrots . . . . .3 quarts Boiling water. . . . . .1 quart Salt . . . . .1½ teaspoons			2. Add carrots to boiling salted water; cook 15 minutes or until tender. Drain well.
Margarine . . . . .½ cup (4 ounces)			3. Combine peas, carrots and margarine; serve hot.

YIELD
50 portions (about 1½ gallons)

PORTION SIZE
½ cup (3 to 4 ounces)

PAN SIZE
Heavy 3-gallon stock pot

VARIATION
Creamed peas and carrots: Use 2 quarts thin cream sauce made with ½ cup all-purpose flour, ½ cup margarine, ½ teaspoon salt and 2 quarts of milk instead of butter or margarine in step 3.

NOTE
1 No. 10 can of peas, simmered in their own juice for 10 to 12 minutes and then drained, may be used instead of frozen peas in step 1.

DIETARY INFORMATION
May be used as written for general, no added salt, bland, soft, low fat and low cholesterol diets. Diabetic diets — each serving provides 2 vegetable exchanges.

YIELD
50 portions (about 1½ gallons)

PORTION SIZE
½ cup (4 ounces)

PAN SIZE
Heavy 3-gallon stock pot

VARIATION
Peas and onions: Use 1½ quarts chopped onions instead of mushrooms in step 2.

NOTE
2 No. 10 cans of peas simmered 10 to 12 minutes in their own juice and then drained well, may be used instead of the frozen peas in step 1.

DIETARY INFORMATION
May be used as written for general, no added salt, bland and low cholesterol diets. Diabetic diets — each serving provides ½ bread exchange.

Peas and Mushrooms

Refer to footnotes for special dietary information

INGREDIENTS	WEIGHTS/MEASURES	YIELD ADJUST.	METHOD
Frozen peas . . . . .10 pounds Salt . . . . .1 tablespoon Boiling water. . . . . .3 quarts			1. Add peas to boiling salted water; simmer 15 to 20 minutes or until peas are tender; drain well.
Canned, drained mushrooms. .2 1-pound cans Margarine . . . . .½ cup (4 ounces)			2. Fry mushrooms in margarine for about 2 minutes; add mushrooms and fat to peas and mix lightly. Serve hot.

Savory Peas and Rice

Refer to footnotes for special dietary information

INGREDIENTS	WEIGHTS/MEASURES	YIELD ADJUST.	METHOD
Long grain rice . . . . .1 pound (2⅓ cups) Cold water. . . . . .4½ cups Salt .1 tablespoon			1. Combine rice, cold water and salt in pot; bring to a boil, stirring occasionally; cover tightly; simmer 15 minutes. Do not stir. If rice is not tender, cover and simmer 2 to 3 minutes longer. Uncover rice; allow it to dry and fluff for 3 to 5 minutes.
Chopped onions . . . . .3 cups Finely chopped celery . . . . . . .3 cups Margarine or bacon fat . . . . . . .½ cup			2. Fry onions and celery in margarine or bacon fat until onions are golden.
Canned peas. . . . . .3 quarts (1 No. 10 can)			3. Simmer peas 10 to 12 minutes in their own juice; drain well.
Canned, crushed tomatoes . . .3 quarts (1 No. 10 can) Sugar. . . . . .¼ cup Salt .1½ tablespoons Pepper. . . . . .½ teaspoon			4. Combine tomatoes, sugar, salt and pepper; cook 10 to 12 minutes in a heavy pot; add drained rice, onions, celery and peas; heat to serving temperature.

YIELD
50 portions (about 2¼ gallons)

PORTION SIZE
¾ cup (6 ounces)

PAN SIZE
Heavy 3-gallon stock pot

DIETARY INFORMATION
May be used as written for general diets. Diabetic diets — each serving provides 1 bread exchange. Bland diets — omit pepper. No added salt diets — use margarine, not bacon fat, in step 2.

YIELD
50 portions (about 1½ gallons)

PORTION SIZE
½ cup (3 to 4 ounces)

PAN SIZE
Heavy 3-gallon stock pot

NOTE
Broth from cooking spareribs or ham may be used in step 2 instead of soup base and water.

DIETARY INFORMATION
May be used as written for general diets. Diabetic diets — omit brown sugar. Sweeten to taste with brown-sugar substitute in step 5. Each serving using sugar substitute provides ½ bread exchange.

Braised Sauerkraut

Refer to footnotes for special dietary information

INGREDIENTS	WEIGHTS/MEASURES	YIELD ADJUST.	METHOD
Canned sauerkraut . . . . 1½ gallons (2 No. 10 cans) Chicken soup base . . . . ½ cup Hot water . . . . .as necessary			1. Drain sauerkraut; discard juice. 2. Combine sauerkraut, soup base and enough hot water to cover sauerkraut; simmer 1 hour; drain sauerkraut; discard liquid; save sauerkraut for use in step 5.
Chopped bacon . . . . ½ pound			3. Fry bacon until crisp in stock pot. Remove bacon from fat with a slotted spoon and keep bacon for use in step 5.
Chopped onions . . . . .3 cups			4. Fry onions in bacon fat until golden.
Brown sugar . . . . .1 cup All-purpose flour . . . . ½ cup			5. Add sauerkraut and bacon to fried onions; mix sugar and flour together; sprinkle over sauerkraut. Cook and stir over moderate heat until flour and sugar are absorbed and sauerkraut is hot.

Baked Butternut Squash

Refer to footnotes for special dietary information

INGREDIENTS	WEIGHTS/MEASURES	YIELD ADJUST.	METHOD
Butternut squash . . . . .16 pounds Salt . . . . .2 tablespoons			1. Cut squash in half; remove seeds and fiber; sprinkle inside of squash with salt; turn upside down on heavily buttered sheet pan. 2. Bake 1½ hours or until skin is slightly browned and squash feels soft to the touch. 3. Cut in serving-size portions and serve hot.

YIELD
50 portions

PORTION SIZE
About ½ cup
(about 4½ ounces)

PAN SIZE
18 × 26-inch sheet pans

TEMPERATURE
375°F. Oven

VARIATIONS
1. Baked cubed squash: Clean squash and cut it in about 1-inch cubes. Put squash in heavily buttered roasting pan; sprinkle with ½ cup brown sugar, 2 teaspoons salt and 2 cups (1 pound) melted butter or margarine. Bake about 1½ hours or until tender, stirring a couple of times during baking time.
2. Mashed winter squash: Clean and cube squash and boil for 20 to 30 minutes in enough water to cover the squash. Drain well and mash with 1 pound butter or margarine, 2 teaspoons salt and 1 teaspoon pepper, adding about 1 cup of milk for the proper consistency.

DIETARY INFORMATION
May be used as written for general, no added salt, low fat, low cholesterol, soft diets and bland diets. Diabetic diets — each serving provides 1 bread exchange.

YIELD
50 portions (2 pans)

PORTION SIZE
1/2 cup (No. 8 dipper)

PAN SIZE
12 × 20 × 2-inch steam table pans

TEMPERATURE
350°F. Oven

NOTE
1. Hubbard, acorn or other winter squash may be used instead of butternut squash in above recipe.
2. 1 No. 10 can tomatoes may be drained and used instead of fresh tomatoes in above recipe.

DIETARY INFORMATION
May be used as written for general, no added salt, bland and low cholesterol diets. Diabetic diets — each serving provides 1 bread and 1 fat exchanges.

Butternut Squash Casserole

Refer to footnotes for special dietary information

INGREDIENTS	WEIGHTS/MEASURES	YIELD ADJUST.	METHOD

Butternut squash . . . . .16 pounds
Fresh tomatoes. . . . . .5 pounds
Chopped onions . . . . .2 quarts
Salt . . . . .1 tablespoon
Italian seasoning . . . . .2 tablespoons
Margarine . . . . .1 cup
(8 ounces)
			1. Peel squash; remove seeds and fiber; cut in slices about 1/2- to 1-inch thick.
			2. Peel and clean tomatoes; slice in 1/2-inch slices.
			3. Layer squash, tomatoes and onions in greased pans as follows:
			    layer of squash
			    layer of tomatoes
			    sprinkle with onions and seasonings
			    dot with margarine
			    layer of squash
			    dot with margarine and seasoning
			4. Cover pan tightly with aluminum foil and bake 1 1/2 hours or until squash is tender.
			5. Remove foil and continue to bake another 1/2 hour or until slightly browned.

Creole Summer Squash

Refer to footnotes for special dietary information

INGREDIENTS WEIGHTS/MEASURES	YIELD ADJUST.	METHOD
Chopped onions . . . . .3½ cups Vegetable oil . . . . .¼ cup		1. Fry onions in oil until light yellow.
Sliced, fresh summer squash. .7 pounds, 8 ounces Boiling water. . . . . .2 cups		2. Add squash and water to onions; simmer for 10 minutes.
Canned, drained, crushed tomatoes. . . . . .1¼ quarts Salt . . . . .2 tablespoons Pepper. . . . . .½ teaspoon Minced garlic . . . . .2 cloves Dried parsley. . . . . .2 tablespoons		3. Add tomatoes, salt, pepper, garlic and parsley to squash; cover and simmer another 5 minutes. Serve hot.

VEGETABLES 22

YIELD
50 portions (about 1½ gallons)

PORTION SIZE
½ cup (3 to 4 ounces)

PAN SIZE
Heavy 3-gallon stock pot

NOTE
7 pounds, 8 ounces frozen, sliced summer squash may be used instead of the fresh squash in step 2. Simmer 5 minutes only in step 2.

DIETARY INFORMATION
May be used as written for general, no added salt and low cholesterol diets. For bland diet delete pepper. Diabetic diets — each serving provides 1 vegetable exchange.

237

YIELD
50 portions

PORTION SIZE
½ tomato

PAN SIZE
18 × 26-inch sheet pan

TEMPERATURE
350°F. Oven

DIETARY INFORMATION
May be used as written for general and no added salt diets. For bland diet delete pepper. Diabetic diets — each serving provides ½ vegetable and 1 fat exchanges.

Baked Tomato Halves

Refer to footnotes for special dietary information

INGREDIENTS WEIGHTS/MEASURES	YIELD ADJUST.	METHOD
Fresh ripe tomatoes . . . . .25 medium		1. Wash tomatoes; cut each tomato in half crosswise. Put tomato halves on well-greased sheet pan.
Margarine, melted. . . . . .1 cup (8 ounces) Garlic salt . . . . .2 tablespoons Pepper. . . . . .2 tablespoons Dehydrated parsley. . . . . .3 tablespoons Grated Parmesan cheese . . . . .½ cup		2. Brush cut surface of each tomato half with melted margarine; sprinkle with garlic salt and pepper; sprinkle with dried parsley and cheese, using about ½ teaspoonful of cheese for each tomato half. 3. Bake 35 to 45 minutes or until tomato is tender and lightly browned.

Country-Style Tomatoes

Refer to footnotes for special dietary information

INGREDIENTS	WEIGHTS/MEASURES	YIELD ADJUST.	METHOD
Canned, crushed tomatoes . . . 1½ gallons (2 No. 10 cans) Sugar. . . . . ½ cup Margarine . . . . ½ cup (4 ounces)			1. Combine tomatoes, sugar and margarine in heavy pot; keep 2 cups juice from the tomatoes for use in step 2; heat to boiling.
All-purpose flour . . . . ½ cup Celery salt. . . . . 1 tablespoon (optional) Onion salt . . . . 1 tablespoon			2. Combine flour, celery salt and onion salt; mix with 2 cups juice from tomatoes; add to hot tomatoes; cook and stir until juice is slightly thickened; cover and simmer over low heat, stirring occasionally, about 15 minutes. Serve hot.

YIELD
50 portions (about 1½ gallons)

PORTION SIZE
½ cup (4-ounce ladle)

PAN SIZE
Heavy 3-gallon stock pot

DIETARY INFORMATION
May be used as written for general, no added salt, low fat, low cholesterol, soft and bland diets. Diabetic diets — omit sugar, sweeten to taste with sugar substitute after step 2. Each serving, using sugar substitute, provides 1 vegetable exchange.

YIELD
50 portions (about 1½ gallons)

PORTION SIZE
½ cup (4 ounces)

PAN SIZE
Heavy 3-gallon stock pot
Roasting pan

TEMPERATURE
350°F. Oven

DIETARY INFORMATION
May be used as written for general, no added salt, bland and low cholesterol diets. Diabetic diets — omit sugar. Add sugar substitute to taste at the end of step 2. Each serving, using sugar substitute, provides 1 vegetable exchange.

Scalloped Tomatoes

Refer to footnotes for special dietary information

INGREDIENTS	WEIGHTS/MEASURES	YIELD ADJUST.	METHOD
Chopped onions . . . . .3 cups Margarine . . . . .½ cup (4 ounces)			1. Fry onions in margarine in heavy pot until onions are golden.
Solid pack tomatoes. . . . . . . .1½ gallons or (2 No. 10 cans) Drained crushed, canned tomatoes. . . . . .1½ gallons Sugar. . . . . .½ cup			2. Add tomatoes and sugar to onions; simmer over low heat 3 minutes. (If regular canned tomatoes are used, it will take about 3 No. 10 cans. Drain tomatoes, saving juice for other uses and then follow the rest of recipe.)
Toasted bread cubes. . . . . . . .1½ quarts (1½ pounds) Salt . . . . .1 tablespoon			3. Add bread cubes and salt to tomatoes; mix lightly; pour into roasting pan.
Bread crumbs . . . . .½ cup (2 ounces) Grated Parmesan cheese . . . . .½ cup Margarine . . . . .½ cup (4 ounces)			4. Combine bread crumbs and cheese; sprinkle over tomatoes; dot with margarine; bake about 30 minutes or until lightly browned.

Stewed Tomatoes

Refer to footnotes for special dietary information

INGREDIENTS	WEIGHTS/MEASURES	YIELD ADJUST.	METHOD
Chopped onions . . . . 1 cup Margarine . . . . 1/2 cup			1. Fry onions in fat in heavy pot until onions are golden.
Canned crushed tomatoes . . . . 1 1/2 gallons (2 No. 10 cans) Sugar. . . . . 1/3 cup Salt . . . . 1 tablespoon Pepper. . . . . 1/2 teaspoon			2. Add tomatoes, sugar, salt and pepper to onions; mix well; bring to a boil; simmer, covered, 10 to 12 minutes. Serve hot.

YIELD
50 portions (about 1 1/2 gallons)

PORTION SIZE
1/2 cup (4-ounce ladle)

PAN SIZE
Heavy 3-gallon stock pot

NOTE
3 quarts of toasted bread cubes may be added to tomatoes just before they are served.

DIETARY INFORMATION
May be used as written for general, no added salt, and low cholesterol diets. Diabetic diets — omit sugar. Add sugar substitute to taste in step 2. Each serving, using sugar substitute, provides 1 vegetable exchange. Bland diets — omit pepper. No added salt diets — use margarine in step 1.

Vegetable Lasagna

Refer to footnotes for special dietary information

YIELD
48 servings (2 pans)

PORTION SIZE
1 square

PAN SIZE
Heavy 3-gallon pot
12 × 20 × 2-inch steam table pans

TEMPERATURE
350°F. Oven

VARIATION
Lasagna with meat sauce: Delete vegetables, meatless tomato sauce and mushrooms. Substitute 2 gallons spaghetti sauce with meat in step 4.

DIETARY INFORMATION
May be used as written for general, no added salt, bland and mechanical soft diets. Diabetic diets — each serving provides 2 bread, 1 lowfat milk and 1 high fat meat exchanges.

INGREDIENTS	WEIGHTS/MEASURES	YIELD ADJUST.	METHOD
Frozen sliced vegetable assortments such as broccoli, green beans, mushrooms, carrots, cauliflower, etc.	4 pounds		1. Cook vegetables until crisp-tender according to directions on the package; drain well and set aside for later use.
Ricotta cheese	4 pounds		2. Place ricotta cheese in mixer bowl; add eggs, garlic powder, parsley and Parmesan cheese; mix at low speed only enough to blend; do not beat; set aside for later use. (The cheese mixture should be refrigerated if it isn't to be used for over 1 hour but must be brought back to room temperature before it is used.)
Eggs	3 cups (15-18 medium)		
Garlic powder	4 teaspoons		
Chopped parsley	1/4 cup		
Grated Parmesan cheese	1 cup		
Lasagna noodles	3 pounds		3. Cook lasagna noodles in boiling water, to which salt and oil have been added, according to directions on the package; drain well. Noodles may be kept in cold water until needed, but they should be drained before they are used.
Hot water	3 gallons		
Salt	2 tablespoons		
Vegetable oil	2 tablespoons		
Meatless tomato sauce for spaghetti	1 1/2 gallons (2 No. 10 cans)		4. Mix spaghetti sauce, mushrooms and cooked vegetables together (vegetables should be in bite-size pieces) for use in panning lasagna.
Drained canned mushroom slices and pieces	2 1-pound cans		
Coarsely grated mozzarella cheese	3 pounds		LAYERING INSTRUCTIONS FOR EACH PAN: 1. 1 quart tomato-vegetable mixture spread evenly over the bottom of the pan. 2. 1/6 of the noodles placed flat and in rows on the sauce. 3. 1/2 of the ricotta filling spread over the noodles. 4. 12 ounces of mozzarella cheese scattered over the filling. 5. 1 quart tomato-vegetable mixture spread over the mozzarella cheese. 6. 1/6 of the noodles flat and in rows over the tomato-vegetable mixture.
Grated Parmesan cheese	2/3 cup		
Leaf oregano	2 tablespoons		

Continues on next page

Continued from preceding page

INGREDIENTS	WEIGHTS/MEASURES	YIELD ADJUST.	METHOD
			7. 1 quart of the tomato-vegetable mixture spread evenly over the noodles. 8. 12 ounces mozzarella cheese scattered over the tomato-vegetable mixture. 9. 1 quart of the tomato-vegetable mixture spread evenly over the mozzarella cheese. 10. 1/6 of the noodles placed flat and in rows over the tomato-vegetable mixture. 11. 1 quart of the tomato-vegetable mixture spread evenly over the noodles. 12. 1/3 cup Parmesan cheese spread evenly over the tomato-vegetable mixture. 13. 1 tablespoon oregano sprinkled evenly over the Parmesan cheese. 14. Bake about 1 hour or until top is bubbling and lightly browned. 15. Let lasagna stand at room temperature for 15 to 20 minutes to allow lasagna to firm up before cutting it 4 × 6. Serve hot.

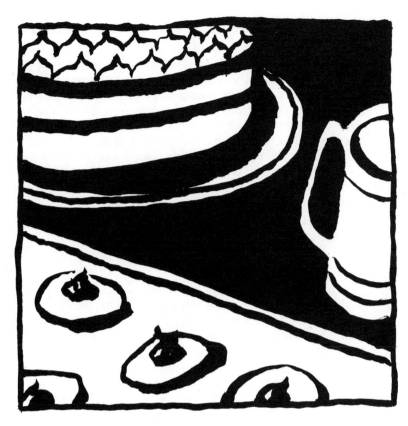

Chapter 11
Cakes and Cookies

Information **246**

Cake and Cookie Information

Cakes and cookies are popular with most residents, and therefore can serve as a valuable source of fiber, calories and nutrients once the basic nutritive needs of the resident have been met. The use of whole-wheat flour, bran cereal, oatmeal, raisins, dates and other fruits can add variety and interest to the cakes and cookies while supplying calories, fiber and some nutrients.

Since fiber is important to most residents, every effort has been made to provide cake and cookie recipes which will appeal to residents as well as supply the fiber which most of them need without reducing the taste appeal because, if the patient doesn't eat the cake or cookie, none of the fiber or other ingredients will be of any use to them. A plain basic cake or cookie generally has very little fiber and therefore it is necessary to add other ingredients to the basic recipe if fiber is to be included in the recipe. Each cake or cookie with a significant amount of fiber has the amount of fiber listed at the bottom of the recipe, along with the other dietary information.

If you want to change the size pans used in these recipes, remember that cakes generally need to have the batter fill the pan about 2/3 fill. The pan size is very important in converting a recipe from one amount to another (see general information for the way to change the amounts in a recipe). One of the easiest ways to do this is to calculate the square inches in the bottom of both pans and then develop the recipe accordingly.

SIZE OF PAN	YIELD IN SQUARE INCHES
9-inch square	81
9-inch round	64
8-inch square	64
8-inch round	50
7 × 11-inch oblong	77
9 × 13-inch cake pan	117
11 × 14-inch pudding pad	154
10 × 12-inch half steam table pan	120
12 × 20-inch steam table pan	240
12 × 18-inch cake pan	216
12 × 18-inch half sheet pan	216
18 × 26-inch full sheet pan	468

After you have established the square inches in a cake pan, you can establish how much the recipe needs to be increased, decreased or how many pans it will fill. Thus, a cake recipe which is right for a 12 × 18-inch cake pan (216 inches) when baked in a 9-inch round pan (64 inches) will yield $216/64 = 3\frac{1}{2}$ or three full layers a little thicker than the original cake, or four layers a little thinner than the original cake. Most food service supervisors would go with the four thinner layers since a layer cake is not generally as thick as a cake baked in a cake pan and cut into squares. Therefore, if you wanted to make four two-layer cakes using 9-inch layer pans, you would double the size of the original recipe.

Note: Do not use Nutra Sweet in menus which call for sugar substitute. Nutra Sweet breaks down in the cooking process.

CAKE PREPARATION

1. Temperature is very important. The oven should be preheated for 10 to 15 minutes before the cake batter is put into the oven to bring the oven to the temperature specified on the package. The door should not be opened until the time specified because every time the oven door is opened, the temperature of the oven falls for a short time.

2. Instructions for mixing and baking should be followed very closely. DO NOT OVERMIX AND DO NOT UNDERMIX. If a mixer is used, the beating time and speed should be followed as closely as possible. If the batter is beaten by hand, a vigorous beating stroke should be used.

3. Pans should be greased and floured if the cake is to be served directly from the pan. If the cake is to be turned out of the pan, it is a good idea to grease the pan and line it with brown paper or regular cake liners. Pans for angel food or chiffon cakes are not greased. Pans should be greased with butter, margarine, lard or shortening. They should not be greased with a strong smelling fat such as bacon fat. Greasing and oiling a pan are two different procedures. If the pan is to be oiled, vegetable oil should be used. If a pan is to be greased, shortening, butter or margarine or lard should be used.

4. Pans should be spaced evenly in the oven to allow the circulation of hot air around them. If only one pan is baked at a time, it should be put in the center of the oven.

5. Instructions regarding baking time should be followed carefully. Cakes should not be removed from the oven until they are thoroughly baked. Batter cakes may be tested by touching the top near the center. If the

indentation remains, the cake is not done and should be baked another 3 to 5 minutes and then tested again. Cakes should not be baked too long because they will be dry and may be burned.

6. Water or other liquid should be measured very carefully. Too little or too much liquid will spoil the proportion of liquid to dry ingredients in the batter and will yield a poor cake.

7. Cakes should be removed from the pans and handled as follows:

BATTER CAKES: Cooled in pan on rack for 10 to 15 minutes. Layer cakes should be removed from the pans onto paper sprinkled with granulated sugar. Sheet cakes may be frosted in the pan or turned out after 10 to 15 minutes onto an inverted pan or brown paper sprinkled with granulated sugar. The cakes should be cooled and then frosted.

ANGEL FOOD OR CHIFFON CAKES: Pans should be inverted to cool cakes. A cup should be put under the corners of the pan if they are not baked in a regular angel food pan. The top of the cake should not be allowed to touch the surface of the counter or cake rack until the cake is cool. After the cake is cool, a knife should be run around the inside of the cake pan and the cake removed and put on an inverted pan or brown paper sprinkled with granulated sugar. Loose crumbs should be brushed off the cake before it is frosted.

COOKIE PREPARATION

1. Cookies are generally composed of the same basic ingredients as cakes. Different types of cookies are made by varying the proportions of the basic ingredients and methods of mixing. Soft cookies have a higher proportion of liquids including eggs and flour. Crisp cookies have a higher proportion of sugar and shortening. A chewy cookie has a higher proportion of sugar and liquid but is lower in fat. Soda is used to make cookies spread and baking powder is used to make them rise. If cookies rise when they should spread out, baking powder may have been unintentionally substituted for baking soda.

2. Cookies should not be baked too long or they will become dry and lose flavor rapidly. Cookies should be served the day they are baked if at all possible to prevent the loss of flavor and texture.

3. Most cookies should be loosened from the baking pan and removed to racks or other pans to cool. Cookies continue to bake if they remain on the hot pans and will generally be difficult to remove if they are allowed to cool on the pans. Cookie dough should be put on cool pans because the dough will spread too much before it is baked if it is put on a hot pan.

4. It is important to follow instructions in the recipe regarding greasing pans. Some cookies require greased pans but other cookies have enough fat in the dough to eliminate the need for greased pans. Pans should never be greased heavily unless the recipe includes directions for heavy greasing because it encourages the spreading of cookie dough. Rancid or strong-flavored fat such as bacon grease should never be used to grease pans for cookies because cookies will pick up the flavors in the fat.

5. For uniform baking, all cookies on a pan should be the same size and thickness and spaced evenly. If less than a full pan of cookies is to be baked, the cookies should be spaced evenly. The use of a level dipper of dough will enable the baker to standardize the size of the cookies more easily and will save time when the cookies are being put on the pans.

6. The use of dippers when placing the cookie dough on sheet pans will yield a more standard size cookie. A No. 40 dipper is equal to $1\frac{1}{2}$ tablespoons dough and a No. 60 dipper is equal to 1 tablespoon dough.

YIELD
54 servings (2 pans)

PORTION SIZE
1 piece

PAN SIZE
12 × 18-inch cake pan

TEMPERATURE
350°F. Oven

DIETARY INFORMATION
May be used as written for general, bland, lactose-free and no added salt diets. Low cholesterol diets — omit eggs. Use 3½ cups liquid egg substitute in step 3.

Apple Date Squares

Refer to footnotes for special dietary information

INGREDIENTS	WEIGHTS/MEASURES	YIELD ADJUST.	METHOD
All-purpose flour	1 quart		1. Place flours, soda, salt and cinnamon in mixer bowl and mix at low speed for about ½ minute to blend well.
Whole-wheat flour	1 quart		
Soda	1½ tablespoons		
Salt	2 teaspoons		
Cinnamon	1½ tablespoons		
Washed cored and diced fresh crisp apples	1 gallon (5 to 6 pounds)		2. Place apples in bowl. Sprinkle with lemon juice. Add dates to apples. Mix lightly and set aside for use in step 4.
Lemon juice	¼ cup		
Chopped dates	3½ cups (1 pound)		
Eggs	3½ cups (18 to 21 medium)		3. Beat eggs, sugar and oil together to blend. Add to flour mixture and beat at medium speed for 1 minute.
Sugar	1½ quarts		4. Add apples and dates to batter. Mix lightly.
Vegetable oil	3 cups		5. Spread ½ of the batter evenly in each of 2 greased and floured cake pans. Bake 45 to 50 minutes or until the cake is firm in the center and pulls away from the sides of the pan. Cool to room temperature.
Powdered sugar (optional)	¼ cup		6. Sprinkle powdered sugar evenly over cakes. Cut each cake 3 × 9.

Chocolate Cake

Refer to footnotes for special dietary information

INGREDIENTS	WEIGHTS/MEASURES	YIELD ADJUST.	METHOD
Sugar	3 cups		1. Place sugar, cocoa, salt and oil in mixer bowl. Mix at medium speed for 1 minute or until very smooth and creamy.
Cocoa	1½ cups		
Salt	1 teaspoon		
Vegetable oil	1½ cups		
Eggs	¾ cup (3 to 4 medium)		2. Add to creamy mixture and mix at medium speed for 1 minute.
Vanilla	1 tablespoon		
All-purpose flour	3½ cups		3. Stir flour and soda together to blend well.
Soda	2 teaspoons		
Water at room temperature	2¼ cups		4. Add water and flour mixture to creamy mixture and beat at medium speed for ½ minute. 5. Pour batter into well-greased cake pan and bake about 30 minutes or until firm in the center and the cake starts to pull away from the sides of the pan. Cool to room temperature.
Frosting	2 cups		6. Spread frosting evenly on cake and then cut 4 × 6.

YIELD
24 servings (1 pan)

PORTION SIZE
1 piece

PAN SIZE
12 × 18-inch cake pan

TEMPERATURE
350°F. Oven

DIETARY INFORMATION
May be used as written for general, soft, bland, no added salt and mechanical soft diets. Low cholesterol diets — omit eggs and use ¾ cup liquid egg substitute in step 2.

YIELD
24 servings (1 pan)

PORTION SIZE
1 piece

PAN SIZE
12 × 18-inch cake pan

TEMPERATURE
350°F. Oven

DIETARY INFORMATION
May be used as written for general, bland, no added salt and low cholesterol diets.

Date Bran Cake

Refer to footnotes for special dietary information

INGREDIENTS	WEIGHTS/MEASURES	YIELD ADJUST.	METHOD
100% Bran, Bran Buds, All Bran or Fiber One . . . . .2 cups Chopped pitted dates . . . . . . .3½ cups (1 pound) Boiling hot water. . . . . .3 cups			1. Place bran, dates and water in mixing bowl. Mix lightly and let sit at room temperature for 30 to 45 minutes. (This timing is very important.)
Sugar. . . . . .2 cups Brown sugar . . . . .1 cup Shortening . . . . .1 cup			2. Place sugars and shortening in mixer bowl. Mix at medium speed until light and fluffy.
Eggs .1 cup (5 to 6 medium) Vanilla. . . . . .1 tablespoon			3. Add eggs and vanilla to creamed mixture and mix at medium speed until creamy. Add bran mixture and mix at medium speed only until well blended.
All-purpose flour . . . . .1 quart Soda .2 teaspoons Baking powder . . . . .2 teaspoons Salt . . . . .2 teaspoons Chopped nuts . . . . .1 cup			4. Stir flour, soda, baking powder and salt together to blend well. Add flour mixture and nuts to creamed mixture. Mix at medium speed until smooth and creamy. Spread evenly in well-greased pan and bake 35 to 40 minutes or until a cake tester comes out clean from the center of the cake. Cool to room temperature.
Lemon or orange-flavored powdered sugar frosting. . . .2 cups			5. Spread frosting evenly on cake and then cut 4 × 6.

Light Applesauce Cake

Refer to footnotes for special dietary information

INGREDIENTS	WEIGHTS/MEASURES	YIELD ADJUST.	METHOD
Shortening . . . . .1 cup Sugar. . . . . .2½ cups			1. Place shortening and sugar in mixer bowl and mix at medium speed until light and fluffy.
Eggs .½ cup (2 to 3 medium) Vanilla . . . . .1 tablespoon			2. Add eggs and vanilla to creamed mixture and beat at medium speed until creamy.
All-purpose flour . . . . .1¼ quarts Soda . . . . .2 teaspoons Baking powder . . . . .1 tablespoon Cinnamon. . . . . .1 tablespoon Salt . . . . .1 teaspoon Applesauce. . . . . .3 cups			3. Stir flour, soda, baking powder, cinnamon and salt together to blend well. Add to creamed mixture along with applesauce and mix at medium speed until smooth.
Washed and drained raisins . . .1 cup Chopped nuts . . . . .1 cup Frosting (optional). . . . . .2 cups			4. Add raisins and nuts to batter and mix lightly. Spread batter evenly in well-greased cake pan. Bake 40 to 45 minutes or until a cake tester comes out clean from the center of the cake. Cool to room temperature. 5. Frost, if desired, and cut 4 × 6.

YIELD
24 servings (1 pan)

PORTION SIZE
1 piece

PAN SIZE
12 × 18-inch cake pan

TEMPERATURE
350°F. Oven

DIETARY INFORMATION
May be used as written for general, bland and no added salt diets. Low cholesterol diets — omit shortening and eggs. Use 1 cup margarine in step 1 and ½ cup liquid egg substitute in step 2.

YIELD
24 servings (1 pan)

PORTION SIZE
1 piece

PAN SIZE
12 × 18-inch cake pan

TEMPERATURE
350°F. Oven

NOTE
This is a firm, European-style cake.

VARIATIONS
1. Raisin spice cake: Add 1 tablespoon cinnamon and 1 teaspoon cloves in step 3. Add 2 cups washed and drained raisins at the end of step 3.
2. Yellow cake: Omit egg whites in step 2. Add 1 cup whole eggs in step 2.
3. Date nut cake: Add 1 cup chopped dates and 1 cup chopped nuts at the end of step 3.
4. Nut cake: Add 2 cups chopped nuts at the end of step 3. Substitute the appropriate flavoring for the almond flavoring in step 2.
5. Chocolate chip cake: Add 2 cups chocolate chips at the end of step 3. Sprinkle 1¼ cups chocolate chips evenly over the top of the cake as soon as it is removed from the oven. Spread the chocolate, after the chips have melted, evenly over the top of the cake. Score the top of the cake 4 × 6 and then cut along those lines after the chocolate has hardened.

DIETARY INFORMATION
May be used as written for general, soft, bland, no added salt and mechanical soft diets. Low cholesterol diets — omit shortening. Use 1¼ cups margarine in step 1.

White Cake

Refer to footnotes for special dietary information

INGREDIENTS	WEIGHTS/MEASURES	YIELD ADJUST.	METHOD
Sugar. .3 cups Shortening . . . . .1¼ cups			1. Place sugar and shortening in mixer bowl. Mix at medium speed until light and fluffy.
Egg whites . . . . .¾ cup (about 6 medium) Vanilla. . . . . .1 tablespoon Almond flavoring . . . . .1 teaspoon			2. Add egg whites, vanilla and almond flavoring to creamed mixture and beat at medium speed about 1 minute or until very creamy.
All-purpose flour . . . . .5½ cups Baking powder . . . . .2 tablespoons Nonfat dry milk . . . . .½ cup Salt . . . . .1 teaspoon Water. . . . . .2¼ cups			3. Stir flour, baking powder, dry milk and salt together to blend well. Add along with water to creamed mixture and beat 1 to 2 minutes at medium speed or until very creamy. 4. Spread dough evenly in greased floured cake pan and bake about 30 minutes or until lightly browned and firm in the center. Cool to room temperature.
Frosting. . . . . .2 cups			5. Spread frosting evenly on cake and cut 4 × 6.

Cheese Cake for Diabetics

Refer to footnotes for special dietary information

INGREDIENTS	WEIGHTS/MEASURES	YIELD ADJUST.	METHOD
Canned unsweetened red sour pitted cherries	1¾ cups (16-ounce can)		1. Drain cherries well, reserving the juice. Add water to the juice, if necessary, to equal 1 cup. Set cherries aside and combine juice and cornstarch. Cook and stir over moderate heat until thickened and clear and the starchy taste is gone. Remove from heat and add flavoring and sugar substitute. Add cherries to the thickened juice, mix lightly and refrigerate until later.
Water	as necessary		
Cornstarch	1 tablespoon		
Almond flavoring	¼ teaspoon		
Sugar substitute	Equal to ¾ cup sugar		
Plain gelatin	3 packets or 2½ tablespoons		2. Stir gelatin and sugar together to blend well. Add boiling water and stir until gelatin is dissolved. Add sugar substitute and lemon juice and set aside for a few minutes until it begins to thicken.
Sugar	2 tablespoons		
Boiling water	1½ cups		
Sugar substitute	Equal to ¾ cup sugar		
Lemon juice	⅓ cup		
Graham crackers	12 2¼-inch crackers		3. Crush graham crackers and place in cake pan along with sugar and melted margarine. Mix to blend and then pat evenly in the bottom of the pan. Set aside until later.
Sugar	3 tablespoons		
Melted margarine	¼ cup		
Part-skim milk ricotta cheese	2 pounds		4. Drain any excess liquid from ricotta but do not press it to remove further liquid. Combine ricotta, vanilla, salt and sugar substitute. Mix lightly until smooth but do not whip it.
Vanilla	2 teaspoons		5. Add the syrupy gelatin mixture with the cheese mixture. Mix lightly until smooth and then pour over the graham cracker crust in the cake pan. Allow the filling to thicken and then pour the cherry mixture evenly over it. Cut 3 × 6.
Salt	½ teaspoon		
Sugar substitute	Equal to ½ cup sugar		

YIELD
18 portions (1 cake)

PORTION SIZE
1 piece

PAN SIZE
9 × 13-inch cake pan

DIETARY INFORMATION
May be used as written for general, bland and mechanical soft diets as well as no added salt diets. Diabetic diets — each portion provides 1 skim milk and 1 fat exchanges.

YIELD
16 portions (1 cake)

PORTION SIZE
1 piece

PAN SIZE
9 × 13-inch cake pan

TEMPERATURE
375°F. Oven

DIETARY INFORMATION
May be used as written for general, bland, no added salt and mechanical soft diets. Diabetic diets — each piece provides 1 bread and 1 fat exchanges.

Chocolate Cake for Diabetics

Refer to footnotes for special dietary information

INGREDIENTS	WEIGHTS/MEASURES	YIELD ADJUST.	METHOD
100% Bran, Bran Buds, All Bran or Fiber One	1½ cups		1. Place bran, water, sugar substitute, eggs, oil, salt and flavorings in mixer bowl. Mix at low speed for ½ minute. Let stand at room temperature for 30 to 45 minutes. (This timing is very important.)
Water	1½ cups		
Sugar substitute	Equal to ½ cup sugar		
Eggs	½ cup (2 to 3 medium)		
Vegetable oil	⅓ cup		
Salt	1 teaspoon		
Chocolate extract (optional)	2 teaspoons		
Vanilla	2 teaspoons		
All-purpose flour	1½ cups		2. Stir flour, baking powder, cocoa, sugar, dry milk and cinnamon together to blend well. Add to bran mixture and mix at medium speed only to blend well. Pour into a well-greased cake pan. 3. Bake 20 to 25 minutes or until firm in the center and the cake pulls away from the sides of the pan. 4. Cool cake to room temperature and cut 4 × 4.
Baking powder	1 tablespoon		
Cocoa	⅓ cup		
Sugar	⅓ cup		
Nonfat dry milk	⅓ cup		
Cinnamon	1 teaspoon		

Genoise Cake for Diabetics

Refer to footnotes for special dietary information

INGREDIENTS	WEIGHTS/MEASURES	YIELD ADJUST.	METHOD
Margarine	¼ cup (2 ounces)		1. Melt margarine and let cool to room temperature. Set aside for use in step 5. 2. Grease pan well with margarine, line with wax paper and grease again with margarine.
Eggs at room temperature	1¼ cups (6 to 7 medium)		3. Place eggs in mixer bowl and mix with a whip at low speed until well blended. Beat at high speed until the batter holds a crease when the whip is removed. (It is very important that the eggs be at room temperature.)
Sugar.	½ cup		
All-purpose flour	1 cup		4. Stir flour, baking powder, sugar substitute and salt together to blend well. Add to egg mixture while beating at low speed. Mix only until flour is absorbed. Do not overmix. 5. Add melted margarine slowly to batter. Do not overmix.
Baking powder	1 teaspoon		
Dry sugar substitute	equal to ⅓ cup sugar		
Salt	½ teaspoon		
Almond or lemon flavoring	1 teaspoon		6. Add flavoring and mix lightly. Pour batter into pan and smooth with a spatula. 7. Bake about 25 minute or until cake is lightly browned and has started to pull away from the sides of the pan. As soon as the cake is removed from the oven, it should be inverted onto a wire rack and the paper removed. 8. Cool cake to room temperature. Cut cake 3 × 4 and use as a basis for shortcake or serve with fruit, gelatin or ice cream.

YIELD
12 portions (1 cake)

PORTION SIZE
1 piece

PAN SIZE
9 × 13-inch cake pan

TEMPERATURE
350°F. Oven

VARIATIONS
1. Chocolate topped cake for diabetics: As soon as the wax paper is removed from the cake, sprinkle the top of the cake evenly with ½ cup miniature chocolate chips. Spread the chocolate evenly over the top of the cake as soon as it is melted. Score the chocolate 4 × 4 to yield 16 portions. Each portion will have the same exchanges as a piece of the basic cake.
2. Chocolate genoise cake for diabetics: Substitute ¼ cup cocoa for ¼ cup of the flour in step 4. The food exchanges remain the same as the basic recipe.

DIETARY INFORMATION
May be used as written for general, bland, no added salt and mechanical soft diets. Diabetic diets — each piece provides 1 bread and 1 fat exchanges.

YIELD
2 1/2 quarts frosting

VARIATIONS
1. Chocolate buttercream frosting: Omit milk in step 2. Add 2 cups cocoa and 1 cup boiling water in step 2.
2. Mocha buttercream frosting: Delete milk in step 2. Add 1/2 cup cocoa and 2/3 cup double-strength very hot coffee in step 2.
3. Lemon buttercream frosting: Delete vanilla in step 2. Add 1 tablespoon lemon flavoring, 2 tablespoons grated lemon rind and 1/4 teaspoon yellow food coloring in step 2.

DIETARY INFORMATION
May be used as written for general, soft, bland, no added salt and mechanical soft diets.

Buttercream Frosting

Refer to footnotes for special dietary information

INGREDIENTS	WEIGHTS/MEASURES	YIELD ADJUST.	METHOD
Butter or margarine.	3 cups (1 pound, 8 ounces)		1. Cream butter or margarine at medium speed until light and fluffy.
Powdered sugar . . . . Salt . . . . Milk . . . . Vanilla	3 1/2 quarts (4 pounds) 1 teaspoon 1/2 cup 2 tablespoons		2. Stir powdered sugar and salt together to blend well and remove any lumps from the sugar. Add along with milk and vanilla to creamed butter or margarine. Beat at medium speed until smooth and creamy. (This frosting freezes well but should be brought back to room temperature before it is used.)

Chocolate Fudge Frosting

Refer to footnotes for special dietary information

INGREDIENTS	WEIGHTS/MEASURES	YIELD ADJUST.	METHOD
Butter or margarine, softened .1 cup (2 sticks) Powdered sugar . . . . .2 pounds (1¾ quarts) Salt .½ teaspoon Cocoa . . . . .1 cup Vanilla . . . . .1 tablespoon			1. Put butter or margarine, sugar, salt, cocoa and vanilla in mixer bowl.
Light corn syrup . . . . .½ cup Hot water . . . . .¼ cup			2. Combine syrup and water; heat to simmering but do not boil; add to ingredients in mixer bowl; beat at low speed 3 to 4 minutes or until smooth. 3. Spread frosting on cool cake. (The frosting will spread if it is cool but it won't be as glossy as it will be if you spread it when it is warm.)

YIELD
1¼ quarts (frosts 1 sheet cake, 6 dozen cupcakes or 3 2-layer cakes)

VARIATIONS
1. Chocolate nut fudge frosting: Add 2 cups chopped nuts to frosting after step 2.
2. Chocolate rum frosting: Add 1 tablespoon rum flavoring to frosting with vanilla in step 1.

DIETARY INFORMATION
May be used as written for general, no added salt, bland, soft, mechanical soft and restricted residue diets.

YIELD
1¼ quarts (frosts 1 sheet cake,
6 dozen cupcakes or 3 2-layer cakes)

VARIATIONS
1. Chocolate frosting: Add ¼ cup cocoa in step 2 and use about ½ cup boiling water instead of the ¼ to ⅓ cup water in step 2.
2. Orange frosting: Omit dry milk, water and vanilla in step 2. Use 2 tablespoons grated orange rind and ⅓ cup orange juice in step 2.

DIETARY INFORMATION
May be used as written for general, soft, bland, no added salt and mechanical soft diets.

Powdered Sugar Frosting

Refer to footnotes for special dietary information

INGREDIENTS	WEIGHTS/MEASURES	YIELD ADJUST.	METHOD
Butter or margarine..........1 cup (8 ounces)			1. Cream butter or margarine in mixer bowl until soft and creamy, using beater at medium speed.
Powdered sugar ....2 pounds 1¾ quarts) Salt ....½ teaspoon Nonfat dry milk.............¼ cup Vanilla....................1 tablespoon Water.....................¼ to ⅓ cup			2. Sift sugar, salt and dry milk together; add to creamed fat; add vanilla; add water while beating at slow speed; scrape down bowl; beat another minute at low speed or until frosting has the desired consistency. 3. Spread frosting on cool cake.

Cereal Cookies

Refer to footnotes for special dietary information

INGREDIENTS	WEIGHTS/MEASURES	YIELD ADJUST.	METHOD
Sugar. .2 cups Brown sugar . . . . .2 cups Margarine . . . . .2 cups (1 pound)			1. Place sugars and margarine in mixer bowl. Mix at medium speed until light and fluffy.
Eggs .1 cup (5 to 6 medium) Vanilla. . . . . .2 teaspoons			2. Add eggs and vanilla to creamed mixture. Mix at medium speed until creamy again.
All-purpose flour . . . . .1 quart Baking powder . . . . .2 teaspoons Soda .2 teaspoons			3. Stir flour, baking powder and soda together to blend. Add to creamed mixture and mix at medium speed only until flour is moistened.
Rolled oats . . . . .1 quart Bran flakes . . . . .2 cups Coconut, chopped nuts, raisins or chocolate chips . . . . .2 cups			4. Add oatmeal, bran flakes and coconut or alternate to dough. Mix at medium speed to blend into dough. Drop, using No. 40 dipper (1½ tablespoons) onto sheet pans which have been lightly greased or sprayed with pan spray. 5. Bake 10 to 15 minutes or until lightly browned. Remove from hot sheet pans to wire rack and cool to room temperature.

YIELD
6 dozen cookies

PORTION SIZE
1 cookie

PAN SIZE
18 × 26-inch sheet pans

TEMPERATURE
375°F. Oven

DIETARY INFORMATION
May be used as written for general, bland and no added salt diets. Low cholesterol diets — omit eggs. Use 1 cup liquid egg substitute in step 2.

YIELD
6 dozen cookies

PORTION SIZE
1 cookie

PAN SIZE
18 × 26-inch sheet pans

TEMPERATURE
350°F. Oven

DIETARY INFORMATION
May be used as written for general, bland and no added salt diets. Low cholesterol diets — omit eggs. Use 1¼ cups liquid egg substitute in step 1. Do not use chocolate chips.

Chocolate Bran Drop Cookies

Refer to footnotes for special dietary information

INGREDIENTS	WEIGHTS/MEASURES	YIELD ADJUST.	METHOD
100% Bran, Bran Buds, All Bran or Fiber One ....3 cups Water.....................¾ cup Eggs ....1¼ cups (6 to 7 medium) Vegetable oil ....1 cup Vanilla....................1 tablespoon Chocolate extract (optional) ...1 tablespoon Vinegar ....1 tablespoon			1. Place bran, water, eggs, oil, vanilla, extract and vinegar in mixer bowl. Mix lightly and let stand at room temperature for 30 to 45 minutes. (This timing is very important.)
All-purpose flour............3 cups Cocoa ....¾ cup Nonfat dry milk.............⅓ cup Baking powder ....1 teaspoon Soda ....1 teaspoon Sugar.....................1½ cups Salt ....1 teaspoon			2. Stir flour, cocoa, dry milk, baking powder, soda, sugar and salt together to blend. Add to bran mixture and mix at medium speed only until flour is moistened.
Chocolate chips, raisins, chopped dates or chopped nuts..................2 cups			3. Add chocolate chips or alternates to dough. Mix only to incorporate into dough. 4. Drop by No. 40 dipper (1½ tablespoons) onto sheet pans which have been lightly greased or sprayed with pan spray. Bake about 10 minutes or until firm. Do not overbake. Remove from hot sheet pans to wire rack to cool to room temperature.

Chocolate Brownies

Refer to footnotes for special dietary information

INGREDIENTS	WEIGHTS/MEASURES	YIELD ADJUST.	METHOD
Sugar . . . . 3 cups Shortening . . . . 2 cups Cocoa . . . . 1 cup All-purpose flour . . . . 3 cups Eggs . . . . 1 cup (5 to 6 medium) Salt . . . . ½ teaspoon Vanilla . . . . 1 tablespoon Water . . . . ¼ cup			1. Place the sugar, shortening, cocoa, flour, eggs, salt, vanilla and water in the mixer bowl in the order listed. Beat 2 minutes at moderate speed, scraping down the bowl twice during the beating period.
Chopped nuts, dates or raisins. 1 cup			2. Add nuts or alternates to dough. Spread evenly in well-greased pan. 3. Bake 25 to 30 minutes or until slightly firm in the center. Do not overbake. 4. Cut 6 × 6 while the brownies are still slightly warm. They may be frosted with butter cream frosting or dusted with powdered sugar, if desired.

YIELD
36 brownies (1 pan)

PORTION SIZE
1 brownie

PAN SIZE
12 × 18-inch sheet pan

TEMPERATURE
350°F. Oven

DIETARY INFORMATION
May be used as written for general, bland and no added salt diets. Low cholesterol diets — omit shortening and eggs. Use 2 cups (1 pound) margarine and 1 cup liquid egg substitute in step 1.

YIELD
36 bars (1 pan)

PORTION SIZE
1 bar

PAN SIZE
12 × 18-inch sheet pans

TEMPERATURE
350°F. Oven

DIETARY INFORMATION
May be used as written for general, bland and no added salt diets. Low cholesterol diets — omit eggs. Use ½ cup liquid egg substitute in step 2.

Chocolate Chip Bars

Refer to footnotes for special dietary information

INGREDIENTS	WEIGHTS/MEASURES	YIELD ADJUST.	METHOD
Margarine at room temperature	1½ cups (12 ounces)		1. Place margarine and sugars in mixer bowl and mix at medium speed until light and fluffy.
Sugar	1 cup		
Brown sugar	1 cup		
Eggs	½ cup (2 to 3 medium)		2. Add eggs and vanilla to creamed mixture and mix at medium speed until creamy.
Vanilla	2 teaspoons		
All-purpose flour	3 cups		3. Stir flour, baking powder and salt together to blend well. Add to creamed mixture and mix at medium speed only until all flour is moistened.
Baking powder	1½ teaspoons		
Salt	1 teaspoon		
Chocolate chips	2 cups (12 ounces)		4. Add chocolate chips to dough. Mix at medium speed only to blend the chips into the dough. Spread the dough evenly in a well-greased pan.
			5. Bake 20 to 25 minutes or until the center is firm and the bars pull away from the sides of the pan. Cut 6 × 6 while the bars are still slightly warm.

Chocolate Chip Cookies

Refer to footnotes for special dietary information

INGREDIENTS	WEIGHTS/MEASURES	YIELD ADJUST.	METHOD
Shortening . . . . .2 cups Sugar. . . . . .1 cup Brown sugar . . . . .1 cup			1. Place shortening and sugars in mixer bowl and mix at medium speed until light and fluffy.
Eggs .1 cup (5 to 6 medium) Vanilla. . . . . .1 tablespoon			2. Add eggs and vanilla to creamed mixture and mix at medium speed to blend.
All-purpose flour . . . . .4¼ cups Soda .2 teaspoons Salt .1 teaspoon			3. Stir flour, soda and salt together to blend. Add to creamed mixture and mix at medium speed until flour is absorbed.
Chocolate chips . . . . .2 cups (12 ounces)			4. Add chocolate chips to dough. Mix at medium speed only until chips are mixed into the dough. 5. Drop, using No. 40 dipper (1½ tablespoons), onto sheet pans which have been lightly greased or sprayed with pan spray. 6. Bake 12 to 15 minutes or until cookies are lightly browned. Remove cookies from hot pans onto wire racks to cool to room temperature.

YIELD
5 dozen cookies

PORTION SIZE
1 cookie

PAN SIZE
18 × 26-inch sheet pans

TEMPERATURE
350°F. Oven

DIETARY INFORMATION
May be used as written for general, bland and no added salt diets. Low cholesterol diets — omit shortening, eggs and chocolate chips. Use 2 cups margarine in step 1, 1 cup liquid egg substitute in step 2 and 2 cups chopped nuts, dates or raisins in step 4.

YIELD
6 dozen cookies

PORTION SIZE
1 cookie

PAN SIZE
18 × 26-inch sheet pans

TEMPERATURE
375°F. Oven

DIETARY INFORMATION
May be used as written for general, bland, restricted bland, no added salt and mechanical soft diets. Low cholesterol diets — omit eggs. Use ¾ cup liquid egg substitute in step 2.

Drop Sugar Cookies

Refer to footnotes for special dietary information

INGREDIENTS	WEIGHTS/MEASURES	YIELD ADJUST.	METHOD
Sugar	1½ cups		1. Place sugar, powdered sugar, margarine and oil in mixer bowl. Mix at medium speed until thick and creamy.
Powdered sugar	1½ cups		
Margarine	1½ cups (12 ounces)		
Vegetable oil	1½ cups		
Eggs	¾ cup (3 to 4 medium)		2. Add eggs and vanilla to creamy mixture. Beat at medium speed until thick and creamy again.
Vanilla	1 tablespoon		
All-purpose flour	1¾ quarts		3. Stir flour, soda and cream of tartar together to blend. Add to creamed mixture and mix at medium speed about ½ minute or until blended.
Soda	1½ teaspoons		4. Drop by No. 40 dipper (1½ tablespoons) onto sheet pans which have been lightly greased or sprayed with pan spray.
Cream of tartar	1½ teaspoons		5. Bake about 12 minute or until lightly browned. Remove from hot sheet pans onto wire racks to cool to room temperature.

Oatmeal Cookies

Refer to footnotes for special dietary information

INGREDIENTS	WEIGHTS/MEASURES	YIELD ADJUST.	METHOD
Margarine . . . . .2 cups (1 pound) Sugar. . . . . .2 cups Brown sugar . . . . .2 cups			1. Place margarine and sugars in mixer bowl and mix at medium speed until light and fluffy.
Eggs .1 cup (5 to 6 medium) Vanilla. . . . . .1 tablespoon			2. Add eggs and vanilla to creamed mixture and mix at medium speed until creamy again.
All-purpose flour. . . . . .1¼ quarts Soda .1 teaspoon Baking powder . . . . .2 teaspoons Salt . . . . .1 teaspoon			3. Stir flour, soda, baking powder and salt together to blend. Add to creamed mixture and mix at medium speed to blend.
Rolled oats . . . . .2 cups Raisins, dates, chopped nuts or chocolate chips . . . . .2 cups			4. Add oatmeal and raisins or alternates to dough and mix at medium speed to blend. 5. Drop by No. 40 dipper (1½ tablespoons) onto sheet pan which has been lightly greased or sprayed with pan spray. 6. Bake 12 to 15 minutes or until lightly browned. Remove from hot sheet pans to wire racks to cool to room temperature.

YIELD
6 dozen cookies

PORTION SIZE
1 cookie

PAN SIZE
18 × 26-inch sheet pans

TEMPERATURE
375°F. Oven

VARIATION
Chocolate oatmeal cookies: Use 4½ cups all-purpose flour and ½ cup cocoa in step 3 instead of 1¼ quarts all-purpose flour.

DIETARY INFORMATION
May be used as written for general, bland and no added salt diets. Low cholesterol diets — omit eggs. Use 1 cup liquid egg substitute in step 2. Do not use chocolate chips.

YIELD
10 dozen cookies

PORTION SIZE
1 cookie

PAN SIZE
18 × 26-inch sheet pans

TEMPERATURE
375°F. Oven

VARIATIONS
1. Double peanut cookies: Add 1 quart chopped peanuts to dough at the end of step 3.
2. Peanut butter chocolate chip cookies: Add 1 quart (1½ pounds) chocolate chips to dough at the end of step 3.

DIETARY INFORMATION
May be used as written for general, bland, and no added salt diets. Low cholesterol diets — omit shortening and eggs. Use 2 cups margarine in step 1 and 1 cup liquid egg substitute in step 2.

Peanut Butter Cookies

Refer to footnotes for special dietary information

INGREDIENTS	WEIGHTS/MEASURES	YIELD ADJUST.	METHOD
Sugar	2 cups		1. Place sugars, shortening, oil and peanut butter in mixer bowl and mix at medium speed until creamy and well blended.
Brown sugar	2 cups		
Shortening	2 cups		
Vegetable oil	1 cup		
Smooth or chunky peanut butter	2 cups		
Eggs	1 cup (5 to 6 medium)		2. Add eggs to creamed mixture and mix at medium speed until creamy again.
All-purpose flour	1¾ quarts		3. Stir flour, soda and salt together to blend well. Add to creamed mixture and mix at medium speed until flour is absorbed.
Soda	4 teaspoons		4. Drop, using No. 40 dipper (1½ tablespoons), onto sheet pans which have been lightly greased or sprayed with pan spray. Press cookie dough down with a fork dipped in cold water.
Salt	2 teaspoons		5. Bake about 12 minutes or until lightly browned. Remove from hot sheet pans to wire rack and cool to room temperature.

Pioneer Bars

Refer to footnotes for special dietary information

INGREDIENTS	WEIGHTS/MEASURES	YIELD ADJUST.	METHOD
Water..................2 cups Margarine...............1 cup (8 ounces) Sugar..................2 cups Raisins................2 cups Ground cinnamon..........2 teaspoons			1. Place water, margarine, sugar, raisins and cinnamon in saucepan. Bring to a boil. Remove from heat and cool to room temperature.
All-purpose flour...........1 quart Soda...................2 teaspoons Salt...................1 teaspoon			2. Place flour, soda and salt in mixer bowl and mix at low speed about $1/2$ minute to blend well. 3. Add raisin mixture to flour mixture and beat at medium speed only until creamy. 4. Spread evenly in well-greased pan. Bake 25 to 30 minutes or until cake tester comes out clean from the center and the cake starts to pull away from the sides of the pan. Cool to room temperature.
Powdered sugar frosting......2 cups			5. Spread frosting evenly over cooled bars. Cut 6 × 6 and serve 1 bar per serving.

YIELD
36 bars (1 pan)

PORTION SIZE
1 bar

PAN SIZE
12 × 18-inch cake pans

TEMPERATURE
350°F. Oven

DIETARY INFORMATION
May be used as written for general, bland, low cholesterol, mechanical soft and no added salt diets.

YIELD
7 dozen cookies

PORTION SIZE
1 cookie

PAN SIZE
18 × 26-inch sheet pans

TEMPERATURE
375°F. Oven

DIETARY INFORMATION
Use as written for general, bland and no added salt diets. Low cholesterol diets — omit shortening and eggs. Use 1 cup (8 ounces) margarine in step 1 and 1 cup liquid egg substitute in step 2. Do not use chocolate chips.

Soft Drop Cookies

Refer to footnotes for special dietary information

INGREDIENTS	WEIGHTS/MEASURES	YIELD ADJUST.	METHOD
Shortening . . . . .2 cups White sugar. . . . . .1 cup Brown sugar . . . . .1 cup			1. Place shortening and sugars in mixer bowl and mix at medium speed until light and fluffy.
Eggs .1 cup (5 to 6 medium) Vanilla . . . . .1 tablespoon			2. Add eggs and vanilla to creamed mixture and mix at medium speed for 1 minute.
All-purpose flour . . . . .1½ quarts Nonfat dry milk . . . . .⅔ cups Soda .1 teaspoon Salt . . . . .2 teaspoons Milk . . . . .1½ cups			3. Stir flour, dry milk, soda and salt together to blend. Add, along with the milk, to the creamed mixture. Mix at medium speed to blend.
Raisins, chopped nuts, chocolate chips or chopped dates . . . . .2 cups			4. Add raisins or alternates to dough. Mix lightly. 5. Drop by No. 40 dipper (1½ tablespoons) onto sheet pans which have been lightly greased or sprayed with pan spray. 6. Bake 12 to 15 minutes or until lightly browned. Remove from hot pans to wire rack to cool to room temperature.

Whole-Wheat Oatmeal Cookies

Refer to footnotes for special dietary information

INGREDIENTS	WEIGHTS/MEASURES	YIELD ADJUST.	METHOD
Margarine . . . . .2 cups (1 pound) Sugar. . . . . .1 cup Brown sugar . . . . .2 cups			1. Place margarine and sugars in mixer bowl. Mix at medium speed until light and fluffy.
Eggs . . . . .¾ cup (4 to 5 medium)			2. Add eggs to creamed mixture and mix at medium speed until creamy again.
Whole-wheat flour. . . . . .1 quart Rolled oats . . . . .1¼ quarts Soda . . . . .2 teaspoons Salt .1 teaspoon Pumpkin pie spice . . . . .1 tablespoon			3. Stir flour, oatmeal, soda, salt and pumpkin pie spice together to blend. Add to creamed mixture and mix at medium speed only until flour is moistened. (1 tablespoon cinnamon may be used instead of the pumpkin pie spice, if desired.)
Chocolate chips, raisins or dates. . . . . .2 cups			4. Add chocolate chips or alternates to dough. Mix lightly. Drop, using No. 40 dipper (1½ tablespoons), onto sheet pans which have been lightly greased or sprayed with pan spray. 5. Bake 10 to 12 minutes or until almost firm on top. Remove from hot sheet pans to wire racks to cool to room temperature.

YIELD
6 dozen cookies

PORTION SIZE
1 cookie

PAN SIZE
18 × 26-inch sheet pans

TEMPERATURE
375°F. Oven

DIETARY INFORMATION
May be used as written for general, bland and no added salt diets. Low cholesterol diets — omit eggs. Use 1 cup liquid egg substitute in step 2. Do not use chocolate chips.

YIELD
6 dozen cookies

PORTION SIZE
1 cookie

PAN SIZE
18 × 26-inch sheet pans

TEMPERATURE
375°F. Oven

DIETARY INFORMATION
May be used as written for general, bland and no added salt diets. Diabetic diets — each cookie provides 1 fruit and 1 fat exchanges.

Coconut Cereal Cookies for Diabetics

Refer to footnotes for special dietary information

INGREDIENTS	WEIGHTS/MEASURES	YIELD ADJUST.	METHOD
Margarine at room temperature	1½ cups (12 ounces)		1. Place margarine and sugar in mixer bowl and mix at medium speed until light and fluffy.
Packed brown sugar	1 cup		
Egg whites	⅔ cup (5 to 6 medium)		2. Add egg whites, flavorings, lemon juice and sugar substitute to creamed mixture and mix at medium speed for 1 minute.
Vanilla	2 teaspoons		
Coconut flavoring	2 teaspoons		
Lemon juice	1 tablespoon		
Liquid sugar substitute	Equal to ½ cup sugar		
All-purpose flour	1 quart		3. Stir flour and soda together to blend and add along with Wheaties, coconut and oatmeal to batter. Mix at medium speed only until all flour is moistened.
Soda	2 teaspoons		4. Drop by No. 60 dipper (1 tablespoon) onto sheet pans which have been lightly greased or sprayed with pan spray. Dip a fork or fingers in cold water and press each cookie into a circle about 2½ inches in diameter.
Wheaties cereal	2 cups		5. Bake about 10 minutes or until lightly browned. (It is important that the cookies be lightly browned to develop their flavor.) Remove cookies from hot pans to wire racks to cool to room temperature.
Shredded coconut	3 cups		
Rolled oats	1 cup		

Double Chocolate Cookies for Diabetics

Refer to footnotes for special dietary information

INGREDIENTS	WEIGHTS/MEASURES	YIELD ADJUST.	METHOD
100% Bran, Bran Buds, All Bran or Fiber One . . . . .2 cups Water. . . . . .²/₃ cup Eggs . . . . .1 cup (5 to 6 medium) Vanilla . . . . .2 teaspoons Chocolate extract . . . . .2 teaspoons Vegetable oil . . . . .²/₃ cup Liquid sugar substitute. . . . . . .equal to ¹/₂ cup sugar			1. Place bran, water, eggs, flavorings, oil and sugar substitute in mixer bowl. Mix lightly and let stand at room temperature for 30 to 45 minutes. (This timing is very important.)
All-purpose flour . . . . .1³/₄ cups Cocoa . . . . .¹/₂ cup Instant dry milk . . . . .¹/₄ cup Soda .1 teaspoon Baking powder . . . . .1 teaspoon Sugar. . . . . .¹/₂ cup			2. Stir flour, cocoa, dry milk, soda, baking powder and sugar together to blend well. Add to bran mixture and mix at medium speed only until flour is moistened.
Miniature chocolate chips . . . .1 cup (6 ounces)			3. Add chocolate chips to dough. Mix lightly. Drop by No. 60 dipper (1 tablespoonful) onto sheet pans which have been greased lightly or sprayed with pan spray. 4. Bake 8 to 10 minutes or until slightly firm. Remove cookies from hot sheet pans to wire racks to cool to room temperature.

YIELD
4 dozen cookies

PORTION SIZE
1 cookie

PAN SIZE
18 × 26-inch sheet pans

TEMPERATURE
350°F. Oven

DIETARY INFORMATION
May be used as written for general, bland and no added salt diets. Diabetic diets — each cookie, when the recipe is used as written, provides ²/₃ bread and 1 fat exchanges. If the chocolate chips are not used, provides ¹/₂ bread and 1 fat exchanges.

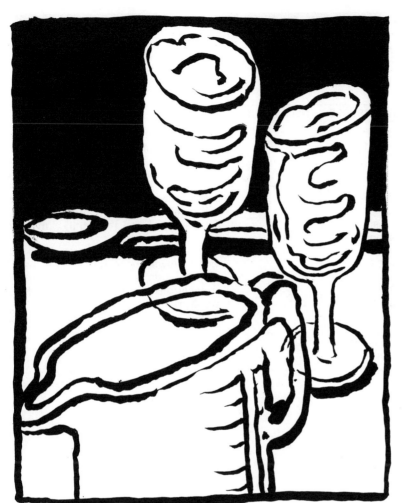

Chapter 12
Puddings

YIELD
50 portions (2 pans)

PORTION SIZE
1/2 cup (No. 8 dipper)

PAN SIZE
12 × 20 × 2-inch steam table pans

TEMPERATURE
375°F. Oven

DIETARY INFORMATION
May be used as written for general, no added salt, low cholesterol, bland and soft diets.

Apple Crisp

Refer to footnotes for special dietary information

INGREDIENTS	WEIGHTS/MEASURES	YIELD ADJUST.	METHOD
Canned drained apple slices . .4½ quarts (1½ No. 10 cans)			1. Arrange half (2¼ quarts) of the apples in each of 2 buttered steam table pans.
Lemon juice . . . . .¼ cup			2. Sprinkle lemon juice over canned apples.
Brown sugar . . . . .3 cups Cornstarch . . . . .½ cup Ground cinnamon. . . . . .1 tablespoon Salt . . . . .2 teaspoons			3. Mix brown sugar, cornstarch, cinnamon and salt together; sprinkle half of the mixture over apples in each pan; mix lightly with apples.
Brown sugar . . . . .1 quart All-purpose flour . . . . .2 cups Rolled oats . . . . .1 quart Baking powder . . . . .1 teaspoon Baking soda . . . . .1 teaspoon Salt . . . . .1 teaspoon Margarine, softened . . . . .1½ cups (12 ounces)			4. Mix brown sugar, flour, rolled oats, baking powder, soda, salt and margarine to form a crumbly mixture; sprinkle half of the mixture evenly over apples in each pan. 5. Bake 40 minutes or until top is browned.

Baked Apples

Refer to footnotes for special dietary information

INGREDIENTS	WEIGHTS/MEASURES	YIELD ADJUST.	METHOD
Baking apples (preferably Rome Beauty) . . . . .50 medium			1. Wash and core apples; pare each apple about ¼ of the way down from top; put apples in shallow baking pan with the pared side up.
Sugar. . . . . .2 quarts Hot water . . . . .3 cups Salt . . . . .1 teaspoon Cinnamon . . . . .1 tablespoon Margarine, melted. . . . . .¼ cup (2 ounces)			2. Combine sugar, water, salt, cinnamon and margarine; stir over low heat until sugar is dissolved and syrup is hot; pour syrup over apples. 3. Bake, uncovered, about 1 to 1½ hours or until apples are tender. (Length of time will depend upon size and kind of apples used.) Baste apples 3 or 4 times while they are baking, using syrup in pan.

YIELD
50 apples

PORTION SIZE
1 apple

PAN SIZE
Shallow baking pan

TEMPERATURE
350°F. Oven

DIETARY INFORMATION
May be used as written for general, no added salt, low fat, low cholesterol and bland diets. Diabetic diets — omit sugar. Use sugar substitute to taste in step 2. Each serving, using sugar substitute, provides 1 fruit exchange. Soft diets — peel apples completely in step 1.

YIELD
2 pans

PAN SIZE
10 × 12 × 2-inch half steam table pans

TEMPERATURE
325°F. Oven

VARIATIONS
1. Caramel custard: Reduce milk to 3¾ quarts; add 1 cup dark Karo syrup with the milk in step 3.
2. Coconut custard: Sprinkle 1 cup of shredded coconut in bottom of each pan before adding custard to be baked.
3. Grapenut custard: Do not use nutmeg in step 4; sprinkle each pan of custard with ½ cup of Grapenuts before it is put in oven.
4. Maple custard: Do not use sugar in step 2; add 2 cups maple syrup and 1 tablespoon of maple flavoring in step 2.
5. Rice custard: Add 2 cups of cooked rice to each pan of custard before sprinkling it with nutmeg in step 4.

DIETARY INFORMATION
May be used as written for general, no added salt, soft and mechanical soft diets. Diabetic diets — omit sugar. Use sugar substitute to taste in step 2. Each serving, using sugar substitute, provides ½ whole milk exchange. Bland diets — omit nutmeg.

Baked Custard

Refer to footnotes for special dietary information

INGREDIENTS	WEIGHTS/MEASURES	YIELD ADJUST.	METHOD
Whole eggs	3 cups (15-18 medium)		1. Put eggs in mixer bowl; mix at low speed, using beater, 1 minute or until well blended but not whipped.
Sugar Salt Vanilla	2 cups 1 teaspoon 1 tablespoon		2. Add sugar, salt and vanilla to eggs; beat 1 minute at low speed or until well blended.
Whole milk Ground nutmeg	1 gallon 1 teaspoon		3. Scald milk by heating it over low heat in a heavy saucepan until small bubbles form around the edge; DO NOT BOIL MILK. Pour hot milk slowly into egg mixture, beating at low speed. 4. Pour half of the mixture (about 2½ quarts) into each of 2 half steam table pans; sprinkle with nutmeg. Put each half pan in a full steam table pan, turning the half pan lengthwise. Put pans in oven and then pour hot water around outside of half pans of custard. 5. Bake 45 minutes to 1 hour or until a knife blade inserted in center of custard comes out clean. 6. Remove pans of custard from the pans of hot water and cool slightly; refrigerate until served.

Cherry Cake Pudding

Refer to footnotes for special dietary information

INGREDIENTS	WEIGHTS/MEASURES	YIELD ADJUST.	METHOD
Margarine, melted	½ cup (1 stick)		1. Spread margarine evenly over bottom of a steam table pan.
Cake flour . . . . Sugar . . . . Nonfat dry milk . . . . Baking powder . . . . Salt	3 cups 3½ cups 1 cup 1 tablespoon ½ teaspoon		2. Sift flour, sugar, dry milk, baking powder and salt together into mixing bowl.
Water	2¾ cups		3. Add water to flour mixture; stir only until well blended; spread batter evenly in buttered pan.
Pitted, red sour cherries	3 quarts (1 No. 10 can)		4. Pour cherries and their juice gently over the batter. (Cherries will sink to the bottom and batter will rise to form a cake layer on top.) 5. Bake about 45 minutes or until lightly browned. 6. Serve in squares with fruit side up.

YIELD
1 pan

PAN SIZE
12 × 20 × 2-inch steam table pan

TEMPERATURE
375°F. Oven

DIETARY INFORMATION
May be used as written for general, no added salt, low fat, low cholesterol, bland and soft diets.

YIELD
48 portions (1 pan)

PORTION SIZE
2 × 2½-inch square

PAN SIZE
12 × 20 × 2-inch steam table pan

TEMPERATURE
350°F. Oven

DIETARY INFORMATION
May be used as written for general and no added salt diets. Bland, soft and mechanical soft diets — omit nuts.

Cocoa Fudge Pudding

Refer to footnotes for special dietary information

INGREDIENTS	WEIGHTS/MEASURES	YIELD ADJUST.	METHOD
Shortening	1½ cups		1. Cream shortening, vanilla and sugar together until light and fluffy.
Vanilla	3 tablespoons		
Sugar	4 cups		
All-purpose flour	5 cups		2. Sift flour, baking powder, salt, dry milk and cocoa together.
Baking powder	4 teaspoons		
Salt	2 teaspoons		
Instant dry milk	¾ cup		
Cocoa	½ cup		
Water	2¼ cups		3. Add flour mixture and water to creamed mixture; mix together about 2 minutes at medium speed or until well blended; scrape down bowl once during mixing period.
Coarsely chopped nuts	3 cups		4. Fold nuts into batter; spread the batter in a well-buttered steam table pan.
Brown sugar	4½ cups		5. Mix sugars, cocoa and salt together; sprinkle over batter.
Sugar	5 cups		
Cocoa	¾ cup		
Salt	2 teaspoons		
Boiling water	2½ quarts		6. Pour boiling water over batter. DO NOT STIR. Bake about 1 hour or until cake layer is firm. (This pudding separates into 2 layers with cake on top and sauce on bottom.) 7. Cut pudding 6 × 8; serve cake on the bottom with sauce on top. This is good served with whipped topping or ice cream.

Easy Peach Crisp

Refer to footnotes for special dietary information

INGREDIENTS	WEIGHTS/MEASURES	YIELD ADJUST.	METHOD
Canned slices peaches ......1½ gallons (2 No. 10 cans)			1. Drain peaches well; spread drained slices evenly in pan.
Cornflake crumbs...........1 quart (12 ounces) Brown sugar ....2 cups Ground cinnamon...........1 tablespoon Margarine, melted..........1 cup (8 ounces)			2. Combine crumbs, sugar, cinnamon and melted margarine; mix thoroughly. Sprinkle crumb mixture evenly over peaches. 3. Bake about 30 minutes or until fruit is heated thoroughly and crumb mixture is crisp. Serve warm or chilled.

YIELD
40 portions (1 pan)

PORTION SIZE
½ cup (No. 8 dipper)

PAN SIZE
12 × 20 × 2-inch steam table pan

TEMPERATURE
400°F. Oven

NOTE
Peach juice may be thickened with cornstarch with a little grated lemon peel and cinnamon added and used as a sauce for the peach crisp.

DIETARY INFORMATION
May be used as written for general, no added salt, low fat, low cholesterol, bland and soft diets. Diabetic diets — omit brown sugar in step 2. Substitute brown sugar substitute to taste. Each serving, using sugar substitute, will provide ½ bread, 1 fruit and 1 fat exchanges.

YIELD
50 portions (about 1½ gallons)

PORTION SIZE
½ cup (No. 8 dipper)

DIETARY INFORMATION
May be used as written for general, no added salt, low fat, bland and soft diets.

Fluffy Fruit Dessert

Refer to footnotes for special dietary information

INGREDIENTS	WEIGHTS/MEASURES	YIELD ADJUST.	METHOD
Canned pineapple chunks or tidbits . . . . .3 quarts (1 No. 10 can) Pineapple juice . . .if necessary			1. Drain the pineapple well; save 3 cups juice for use in step 2; add canned pineapple juice if necessary for a total of 3 cups.
Sugar. . . . . .⅔ cup Cornstarch . . . . .⅔ cup			2. Mix sugar and cornstarch; add to pineapple juice; stir until smooth. Cook and stir over moderate heat until smooth and thickened. 3. Add drained pineapple to sauce; cool to lukewarm.
Fresh bananas . . . . .2 pounds Drained canned mandarin oranges or diced canned drained peaches . . . . .1 quart Chopped drained maraschino cherries. . . . . .½ cup			4. Peel and slice bananas; add with oranges or peaches and cherries to pineapple mixture.
Dehydrated topping mix . . . . . .8 ounces Miniature marshmallows . . . . .3 cups			5. Prepare dehydrated topping mix according to directions on package; add marshmallows; fold into the fruit mixture. Chill well before serving.

Fruit Cobblers

Refer to footnotes for special dietary information

INGREDIENTS	WEIGHTS/MEASURES	YIELD ADJUST.	METHOD
Canned fruit . . . . 1½ gallons (2 No. 10 cans)			1. Drain fruit well; keep juice for use in step 2.
Lemon juice . . . . ¾ cup Sugar. . . . . 2 to 4 cups Cornstarch . . . . 1¾ cups Salt . . . . 1½ teaspoons			2. Add lemon juice, sugar, cornstarch and salt to cold juice. (The amount of sugar needed will depend upon the kind of fruit used.) Mix until smooth. 3. Cook and stir fruit juice mixture over moderate heat until clear and thickened; add drained fruit; mix lightly; pour half of the fruit mixture into each of 2 steam table pans.
BISCUIT TOPPING: Biscuit mix . . . . 2 pounds, 8 ounces Sugar. . . . . ⅓ cup Margarine . . . . ¾ cup (1½ sticks) Water. . . . . 2 cups			1. Blend ingredients together; do not overmix. Drop dough by tablespoonfuls onto hot fruit mixture. 2. Bake 25 minutes or until topping is lightly browned.
CAKE TOPPING: White or yellow cake mix . . . . . 2 pounds, 8 ounces NOTE: Use biscuit or cake topping.			1. Prepare cake mix according to directions on package; pour ½ of the batter on top of hot fruit in each pan. 2. Bake about 25 to 30 minutes or until the cake is firm in the center and lightly browned.

YIELD
50 portions (2 pans)

PORTION SIZE
½ cup (No. 8 dipper)

PAN SIZE
12 × 20 × 2-inch steam table pans

TEMPERATURE
350°F. Oven

DIETARY INFORMATION
May be used as written for general, no added salt, bland, soft diets.

YIELD
48 portions (2 pans)

PORTION SIZE
3 × 3½-inch square

PAN SIZE
12 × 20 × 2-inch steam table pans

TEMPERATURE
350°F. Oven

DIETARY INFORMATION
May be used as written for general and no added salt diets. Low cholesterol diets — omit eggs. Use 1 cup liquid egg substitute in step 2. Serve without ice cream or topping. A thickened fruit juice or skim milk may be used as a topping. Bland and soft diets — omit nuts.

Fruit Cocktail Pudding

Refer to footnotes for special dietary information

INGREDIENTS	WEIGHTS/MEASURES	YIELD ADJUST.	METHOD
Fruit cocktail..............	3 quarts (1 No. 10 can)		1. Drain fruit cocktail; keep juice for use in step 2.
Sugar................... Sifted all-purpose flour....... Baking soda.............. Salt................... Ground cinnamon.......... Eggs....................	1¾ quarts 1½ quarts 2 tablespoons 2 tablespoons 2 tablespoons 1 cup (5 to 6 medium)		2. Sift sugar, flour, soda, salt and cinnamon together; put in a mixer bowl; add eggs and juice from fruit cocktail. 3. Mix 1 minute at low speed; scrape down bowl; add drained fruit cocktail; mix ½ minute longer at low speed. 4. Put ½ of the batter (about 2½ quarts) in each of 2 well-buttered steam table pans.
Brown sugar.............. Chopped English walnuts .... Ice cream or topping........	2⅓ cups 2 cups as desired		5. Combine brown sugar and walnuts; sprinkle ½ of mixture evenly over each pan of batter. 6. Bake 40 to 45 minutes or until browned. 7. Cut each pan 6 × 4; serve warm or chill and serve with ice cream or whipped topping.

Strawberry Fluff Pudding

Refer to footnotes for special dietary information

INGREDIENTS	WEIGHTS/MEASURES	YIELD ADJUST.	METHOD
Graham cracker crumbs......2 quarts (1 pound) Melted margarine ....½ cup (4 ounces) Sugar....................⅔ cup			1. Combine crumbs, margarine and sugar. Mix well and pat evenly in the bottom of cake pan. Bake 10 minutes. Cool to room temperature.
Strawberry fruit-flavored gelatin..................1 cup (about 7 ounces) Boiling water..............2 cups Fresh or frozen sliced strawberries in sugar ......1 quart (2 pounds)			2. Dissolve gelatin in boiling water. Add frozen strawberries and stir until strawberries are defrosted. Chill until syrupy.
Whipped topping ....3 quarts			3. Prepare whipped topping as directed on the container. Stir syrupy gelatin into the whipped topping while mixing at low speed with whip. Spread evenly in cooled graham cracker crust in pan. Chill until firm.
Fresh or frozen whole strawberries ....24 Whipped topping ....2 cups			4. Cut pudding 4 × 6. Serve garnished with about a tablespoon of whipped topping in which a strawberry has been placed.

YIELD
24 portions (1 pan)

PORTION SIZE
1 square

PAN SIZE
12 × 18-inch cake pan

TEMPERATURE
350°F. Oven

NOTES
1. Other fruits and gelatins may be substituted for the strawberries and strawberry gelatin such as frozen raspberries and raspberry gelatin, blueberries and lemon gelatin or cherries and cherry gelatin.
2. This filling without the crust is an excellent filling for cream puffs. This amount of filling will fill 48 medium-size cream puffs. The cream puffs should be chilled after the filling has been added to them and garnished with whipped topping and a fresh strawberry just before they are served.

DIETARY INFORMATION
May be used as written for general, no added salt and bland diets. Mechanical soft diets — chill filling without crust and strawberry topping.

YIELD
50 portions (about 1½ gallons)

PORTION SIZE
½ cup (No. 8 dipper)

PAN SIZE
Heavy 3-gallon pot

VARIATION NOTE
Fruit tapioca — Add 1 quart drained, chopped fruit to the tapioca after step 3. Since tapioca pudding is not very colorful, it should be garnished with a spoon of jelly, a cube of fruit-flavored plain gelatin, a piece of fruit or a maraschino cherry. You can also sprinkle a little bit of fruit-flavored gelatin to which water has not been added on the top of it for flavor and color.

DIETARY INFORMATION
May be used as written for general, no added salt, bland, soft and mechanical soft diets.

Tapioca Pudding

Refer to footnotes for special dietary information

INGREDIENTS WEIGHTS/MEASURES	YIELD ADJUST.	METHOD
Whole milk . . . . .1 gallon Pearl tapioca . . . . .1½ cups		1. Heat milk to simmering in a heavy pot over low heat; stir tapioca gradually into the milk; simmer 20 minutes, stirring frequently, or until clear.
Slightly beaten egg yolks . . . . .10 Sugar. . . . . .2½ cups Salt . . . . .2 teaspoons Vanilla . . . . .1 tablespoon		2. Mix egg yolks, sugar, salt and vanilla together; add slowly to tapioca, stirring constantly; cook over low heat, stirring frequently, about 10 minutes; remove from heat; cool.
Egg whites . . . . .10 Sugar. . . . . .½ cup		3. Beat egg whites until frothy; add sugar and continue to beat at high speed about 3 minutes to form a meringue. Fold meringue carefully into the tapioca pudding; refrigerate until served.

Whipped Gelatin

Refer to footnotes for special dietary information

INGREDIENTS	WEIGHTS/MEASURES	YIELD ADJUST.	METHOD
Fruit-flavored gelatin. . . . . . . .1 pound, 8 ounces Boiling water. . . . . .2 quarts Cold fruit juice or water. . . . . .2 quarts			1. Dissolve gelatin in boiling water. 2. Add cold fruit juice or water to hot gelatin; stir lightly to mix together. 3. Chill until thickened and syrupy but not firm.
Nonfat dry milk . . . . .1 cup			4. Put gelatin in a chilled mixer bowl; add dry milk; beat at high speed until it keeps its shape. Pour into a steam table pan or individual dishes; chill at least 2 hours.

YIELD
1 pan (2 to 3 gallons)

PAN SIZE
12 × 20 × 2-inch steam table pan

NOTE
1 quart coarsely chopped fruit may be folded into the gelatin after its whipped.

DIETARY INFORMATION
May be used as written for general, no added salt, low fat, low cholesterol, bland, soft and mechanical soft diets. Diabetic diets — substitute diabetic fruit-flavored gelatin for the gelatin in step 1. A serving may be considered free.

YIELD
20 portions (1 pan)

PORTION SIZE
1 square

PAN SIZE
9 × 13-inch cake pan

TEMPERATURE
325°F. Oven

DIETARY INFORMATION
May be used as written for general, no added salt, bland and mechanical soft diets. Diabetic diets — each serving provides 1 lowfat milk exchange. Low cholesterol diets — omit eggs. Use 2 cups liquid egg substitute in step 2.

Pumpkin Custard for Diabetics

Refer to footnotes for special dietary information

INGREDIENTS	WEIGHTS/MEASURES	YIELD ADJUST.	METHOD
Water............3 cups Nonfat dry milk............1½ cups			1. Place water and dry milk in mixer bowl. Mix at low speed to dissolve the milk.
Canned pureed pumpkin.....1 quart Eggs............2 cups (10-12 medium) Molasses............⅔ cup Salt............1 teaspoon Pumpkin pie spice............2 tablespoons Sugar substitute............Equal to 1 cup sugar Diabetic whipped topping (optional)............1¼ cups			2. Add pumpkin, eggs, molasses, salt, spice and sugar substitute to milk. Beat at medium speed about 1 minute or until smooth. Pour into pan and bake about 1¼ hours or until a knife comes out clean from the center of the pudding. 3. Cool to room temperature; refrigerate if not used within an hour. Cut 4 × 5 and serve with 1 tablespoon diabetic whipped topping, if desired.

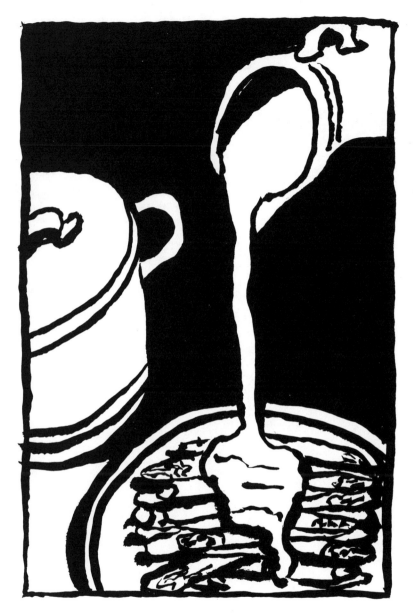

Chapter 13
Sauces

Brown Gravy

Refer to footnotes for special dietary information

YIELD
About 1 gallon

PAN SIZE
Heavy 6-quart saucepan

VARIATIONS
1. Chicken or turkey gravy: Use chicken or turkey fat and broth instead of drippings or shortening and stock, water or drippings.
2. Cream gravy: Do not brown the flour and fat in step 1. Add 1 quart nonfat dry milk to stock, water or drippings in step 2; mix well and then add the flour mixture. DO NOT BOIL the milk before the flour is added.
3. Giblet gravy: Add 3 cuts chopped, cooked giblets to chicken or turkey gravy in step 2.
4. Onion gravy: Brown 1 quart chopped onions in fat before adding flour in step 1.
5. Vegetable gravy: Add 1 quart (1/3 No. 10 can) drained, canned mixed vegetables after step 2.
6. Tomato gravy: Add 3 1/2 cups (1 No. 2 1/2 can) tomato sauce to 3 quarts hot stock and use instead of the stock, water or drippings in step 2.

DIETARY INFORMATION
May be used as written for general, no added salt, bland, soft and mechanical soft diets. Diabetic diets — up to 1/4 cup gravy may be considered free.

INGREDIENTS WEIGHTS/MEASURES	YIELD ADJUST.	METHOD
Fat from meat drippings or shortening. . . . . .1 cup All-purpose flour . . . . .2 cups		1. Melt fat; add flour; cook and stir over low heat until light brown; remove from heat and cool.
Stock, water or drippings or a combination of them . . . . . .1 gallon Salt . . . . .as necessary		2. Put stock, water or drippings in saucepan; add salt to taste; heat to a simmer; add flour mixture, stirring constantly, simmer 10 minutes or until thickened, stirring constantly.

288

Natural Pan Gravy

Refer to footnotes for special dietary information

INGREDIENTS WEIGHTS/MEASURES	YIELD ADJUST.	METHOD
Hot drippings and meat juices .3 quarts Boiling water. . . . . .1 quart		1. Skim any excess fat from meat drippings; add water to drippings; stir and scrape the bottom and sides of roasting pan until drippings, water and brown particles are well blended; measure drippings and pour into saucepan.
Worcestershire sauce. . . . . . . .¼ cup Salt . . . . .1 tablespoon Pepper. . . . . .½ teaspoon		2. Add Worcestershire sauce, salt and pepper to drippings using the amounts given here for 1 gallon hot drippings and meat juices; heat stock over medium heat; serve hot.

YIELD
About 1 gallon

PAN SIZE
Heavy 6-quart saucepan

DIETARY INFORMATION
May be used as written for general, no added salt, low fat, soft and mechanical soft diets. Diabetic diets — remove as much fat as possible from drippings. If almost all of the fat is removed, the gravy may be considered free. Bland diets — omit pepper. Low cholesterol diets — chill drippings and remove fat. Reheat drippings and add 1 cup margarine before proceeding with step 2, if desired, or the pan juices may be served without additional fat.

YIELD
About 1 gallon

PAN SIZE
Heavy 2 or 3-gallon pot

VARIATIONS
1. Cheese sauce: Add 1 pound grated or shredded cheddar or American process cheese after step 2; stir until cheese is melted.
2. Egg sauce: Add 12 chopped, hard-cooked eggs after step 2.
3. Parsley sauce: Add 2 cups finely chopped fresh parsley after step 2.
4. Pimiento sauce: Add 14 ounces (2 7-ounce cans) drained, chopped pimiento after step 2.
5. Fricassee sauce: Use 1 gallon meat or chicken stock instead of the nonfat dry milk in step 1 and the water in step 2.

NOTE
Several methods of making cream or white sauce are used in recipes in this book in order to acquaint users with the different methods. This method is considered to be the simplest and easiest method.

DIETARY INFORMATION
May be used as written for general, no added salt, bland, soft and mechanical diets. Diabetic diets — ⅓ cup of thin white sauce yields 1 vegetable exchange. ⅓ cup of medium white sauce yields ½ bread and ½ fat exchanges. ⅓ cup thick white sauce yields ½ bread and 2 fat exchanges.

Cream or White Sauce

Refer to footnotes for special dietary information

INGREDIENTS	WEIGHTS/MEASURES	YIELD ADJUST.	METHOD
THIN Melted butter or margarine	1 cup (8 ounces)		1. Stir melted butter or margarine, flour, dry milk and salt together to mix very well.
All-purpose flour	1 cup		
Nonfat dry milk	1 quart		
Salt	2 tablespoons		
MEDIUM Melted butter or margarine	2 cups (1 pound)		
All-purpose flour	2 cups		
Nonfat dry milk	1 quart		
Salt	2 tablespoons		
THICK Melted butter or margarine	3 cups (1 pound, 8 ounces)		
All-purpose flour	3 cups		
Nonfat dry milk	1 quart		
Salt	2 tablespoons		
Hot water	3¾ quarts		2. Place water in pot and bring to a boil. Add flour mixture to hot water, stirring constantly with a wire whip. Cook and stir over medium heat until thickened and the starchy taste is gone. (The wire whip is essential. This method will not work unless a whip is used and the sauce is stirred vigorously with the whip.)

Fruit Cocktail Sauce

Refer to footnotes for special dietary information

YIELD
About 1 gallon

PAN SIZE
Heavy 6-quart saucepan

DIETARY INFORMATION
May be used as written for general, no added salt, bland, soft, low fat and low cholesterol diets. Diabetic diets — use fruit cocktail canned without sugar in step 1. Sweeten to taste with sugar substitute at the end of step 3. Using sugar substitute and fruit cocktail canned without sugar, each ¼ cup serving provides ⅓ fruit exchange.

INGREDIENTS	WEIGHTS/MEASURES	YIELD ADJUST.	METHOD
Canned fruit cocktail in heavy syrup	3 quarts (1 No. 10 can)		1. Put fruit cocktail in saucepan; heat to a simmer.
Cold water Cornstarch	1 quart ⅓ cup		2. Combine cornstarch and water; stir until smooth; stir gradually into hot fruit cocktail; cook and stir over moderate heat until thickened and clear and the starchy taste is gone; remove from heat.
Lemon juice Margarine Salt	¼ cup ¼ cup (2 ounces) 1 teaspoon		3. Add lemon juice, butter or margarine and salt to hot sauce; stir lightly to mix; serve hot.

YIELD
About 1 gallon

PAN SIZE
Heavy 6-quart saucepan

VARIATION
Raisin fruit sauce: Add ¼ cup frozen concentrated orange juice and 2 teaspoons pumpkin pie spice instead of the lemon juice in step 2.

DIETARY INFORMATION
May be used as written for general, no added salt, low fat, low cholesterol and bland diets. Diabetic diets — omit sugar and cut raisins to 2 cups. Using sugar substitute and with only 2 cups raisins, each ¼ cup serving provides ⅓ fruit exchange. Up to 2 tablespoons sauce may be considered free.

Raisin Sauce

Refer to footnotes for special dietary information

INGREDIENTS	WEIGHTS/MEASURES	YIELD ADJUST.	METHOD
Cold water. . . . . .1 quart Cornstarch . . . . .¾ cup Brown sugar . . . . .2 cups Boiling water. . . . . .2 quarts			1. Combine cold water, cornstarch and sugar; mix until smooth; pour slowly into boiling water and cook and stir over moderate heat until thickened and clear; remove from heat.
Lemon juice . . . . .¼ cup Salt . . . . .½ teaspoon Washed and drained raisins . . .1¼ quarts 1⅔ pounds)			2. Add lemon juice, salt and raisins to hot sauce; stir lightly to mix; serve hot.

Seafood Cocktail Sauce

Refer to footnotes for special dietary information

INGREDIENTS	WEIGHTS/MEASURES	YIELD ADJUST.	METHOD
Catsup . . . . .1½ quarts Chili sauce . . . . .1½ quarts Lemon juice . . . . .½ cup Worcestershire sauce. . . . . . .2 tablespoons Prepared horseradish . . . . .¼ cup Finely chopped onions. . . . . . .½ cup Finely chopped celery . . . . . . .1 quart			1. Combine ingredients; mix well and refrigerate until used. (If the sauce is to be held in the refrigerator longer than 4 hours, the celery should be added at the last minute.)

YIELD
About 1 gallon

DIETARY INFORMATION
May be used as written for general, no added salt and low cholesterol diets.

YIELD
About 1¼ gallons

VARIATION
Tangy tartar sauce: Cut pickle relish to 1 cup and add 1 quart finely chopped celery, ¼ cup finely chopped parsley and ¼ cup salad mustard.

DIETARY INFORMATION
May be used as written for general and bland diets. Diabetic diets — use cooked diabetic salad dressing. Each serving of 2 tablespoons, using cooked diabetic salad dressing, provides 1 vegetable exchange. Up to 1 tablespoon serving may be considered free.

Tartar Sauce

Refer to footnotes for special dietary information

INGREDIENTS	WEIGHTS/MEASURES	YIELD ADJUST.	METHOD
Salad dressing . . . . .1 gallon Sweet pickle relish . . . . .1 quart Lemon juice . . . . .1 cup Very finely chopped onions . . .1 cup Salt . . . . .1 tablespoon			1. Put salad dressing in mixing bowl; add remaining ingredients and mix lightly by hand until well blended; refrigerate until used.

Tomato Sauce

Refer to footnotes for special dietary information

INGREDIENTS	WEIGHTS/MEASURES	YIELD ADJUST.	METHOD
Tomato puree . . . . .3 quarts (1 No. 10 can)			1. Combine all ingredients in a heavy saucepan and simmer, uncovered, 25 to 30 minutes over low heat; serve hot.
Finely chopped onions . . . . . . .1 cup			
Finely chopped celery . . . . . . .1 cup			
Finely chopped fresh green peppers . . . . .1/2 cup			
Bay leaf 1			
Basil .1/2 teaspoon			
Salt . . . . .2 teaspoons			
Pepper . . . . .1/2 teaspoon			
Dried parsley flakes . . . . .2 tablespoons			
Margarine . . . . .1/4 cup (2 ounces)			
Water or stock . . . . .2 cups			

YIELD
About 3½ quarts

PAN SIZE
Heavy 6-quart saucepan

DIETARY INFORMATION
May be used as written for general, no added salt and low cholesterol diets. Diabetic diets — each serving of ½ cup provides 2 vegetable exchanges. Bland diets — omit pepper and fresh green peppers.

YIELD
50 portions (about 1½ gallons)

PORTION SIZE
½ cup (No. 8 dipper)

PAN SIZE
Roasting pan

TEMPERATURE
350°F. Oven

VARIATIONS
1. Apple sage dressing: Add 1 quart chopped, drained, canned apples to bread with the celery and onions in step 2.
2. Giblet dressing: Add 3 cups chopped cooked giblets with the celery and onions in step 2.
3. Raisin dressing: Add 1 cup washed and drained raisins with the celery and onions in step 2.

DIETARY INFORMATION
May be used as written for general and no added salt diets. Diabetic diets — ½ cup serving provides 1½ bread and 1 lean meat exchanges. ⅓ cup serving provides 1 bread, ½ lean meat and 1 fat exchanges. Low cholesterol diets — use margarine in step 1. Omit eggs and use 1½ cups liquid egg substitute in step 4. Bland diets — omit pepper.

Bread Dressing

Refer to footnotes for special dietary information

INGREDIENTS	WEIGHTS/MEASURES	YIELD ADJUST.	METHOD
Turkey or chicken fat or margarine . . . . .1 pound (about 2 cups) Finely chopped celery . . . . . . .1½ quarts Finely chopped onions . . . . . . .3 cups			1. Fry celery and onions in fat until onions are light yellow.
Diced day-old white bread . . . .5 pounds (2½ gallons)			2. Pour onions, celery and fat over bread and mix lightly.
Hot water . . . . .3 quarts Chicken-flavored soup and gravy base. . . . . .⅓ cup			3. Stir soup base into water; heat and stir until soup base is dissolved; cool to lukewarm.
Slightly beaten eggs. . . . . .1½ cups (8-9 medium) Salt . . . . .2 teaspoons Pepper. . . . . .1 teaspoon Ground sage . . . . .1½ tablespoons			4. Add eggs, salt, pepper and sage to lukewarm chicken stock; pour over bread mixture; mix lightly but thoroughly; do not overmix. 5. Put dressing in well-greased roasting pan and bake 1½ hours or until top is browned.

Chapter 14
Bread

Information   **298**

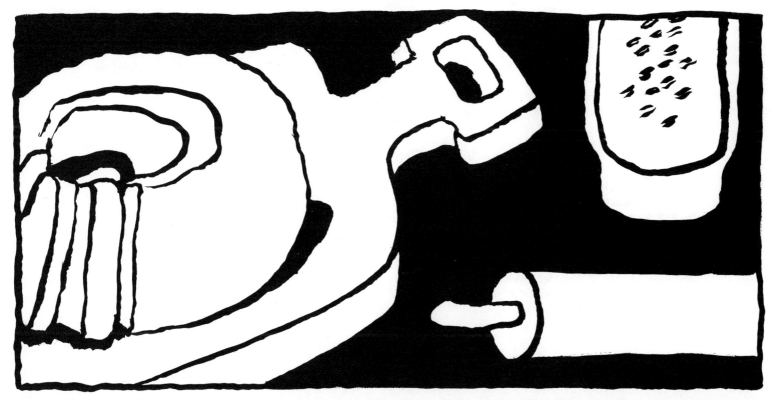

Bread Information

Bread is a basic part of the American diet, and because it is, it can be used to help residents feel more at home in their surroundings. There are many good mixes available as well as frozen doughs which give good results. However, there is still a place for homemade breads in the modern kitchen.

Breads can be a very good source of fiber if prepared correctly, and can be very acceptable to residents as well. Several recipes have been included, with information regarding their fiber content — which are good sources of fiber as well as familiar and tasty.

Preparing yeast and hot breads is not difficult but it does require quality ingredients, attention to recipes and an understanding of techniques and ingredients.

Flour

Most yeast breads are made from bread flour or all-purpose flour because of their higher gluten content. When whole wheat, graham, corn, or rye flours are used in yeast breads, they are generally added after the gluten has been developed in the white flour because of their low gluten content. However, flours are combined and added all at once in hot breads because their leavening is provided by baking soda or baking powder and it is not necessary to develop the gluten.

White flour may be stored in a cool dry place but it is important to refrigerate whole grain flours if not used within a few days to prevent rancidity.

Yeast

Yeast is a living organism which must be kept healthy and alive to rise successfully. Yeast grows best at a temperature of 78°F. to 98°F. but will die at any temperature over 140°F. Active dry yeast may be stored at room temperature for several months but compressed yeast must be refrigerated until it is used and should not be kept over two to three weeks. Compressed yeast should be dissolved in liquid about 85°F. to 87°F., but active dry yeast should be dissolved in liquid about 110°F. to 115°F. Some recipes have been developed in which yeast is not dissolved in water but is added to the flour, and the temperature is controlled by adding hot liquid to the flour.

Liquid

It is important to use the right proportion of liquid in relation to the other ingredients in yeast breads. If too little liquid is used, the dough will be heavy and the yeast won't grow as well. If too much liquid is added, the dough will be sticky, hard to handle, and will probably fall when baked. It is difficult to specify the exact amount of liquid which is perfect for a certain amount of flour because some flours absorb more liquid than others. Therefore, most recipes state a standard amount of liquid and allow a little leeway in the amount of flour used in yeast breads.

Instant Dry Milk

Instant dry milk is used in these recipes because it is convenient and economical. It may be dissolved in water before it is added or it may be combined with dry ingredients. Milk helps soften the texture of yeast breads, gives a browner crust, and helps retain freshness.

Sugar

Sugar provides food for yeast and adds flavor and tenderness to bread. However, a large amount of sugar added to yeast breads will retard the development of the yeast and therefore additional yeast may be necessary in some sweet breads.

Salt

Salt improves the flavor of breads and helps strengthen gluten in yeast breads, but it slows down the action of yeast so it should be added after the yeast has had a chance to develop. Breads made from rye or whole wheat flour or breads high in milk or shortening need more salt.

Baking Soda

Baking soda is a leavening agent which reacts with acids such as lemon juice, vinegar, molasses, sour milk, buttermilk, or sour cream. Many older recipes include directions for dissolving soda in liquid because it was often caked and hard to use, but this is not necessary now because soda is no longer caked and may be added with other dry ingredients.

Baking Powder

Baking powder is a dry leavening agent which is activated by liquid. Therefore, doughs or batters including baking powder should be baked as soon as possible after liquid and dry ingredients are combined unless the recipe states otherwise. Double-action baking powder was used to test recipes in this book.

Vegetable Oil

Vegetable oil is used in recipes in this book because it is convenient, easy to measure, doesn't need to be melted, and yields a good product.

YIELD
48 slices (4 loaves)

PORTION SIZE
1 slice

PAN SIZE
9 × 5 × 3-inch loaf pans

TEMPERATURE
350°F. Oven

DIETARY INFORMATION
May be used as written for general, no added salt, bland, soft and mechanical soft diets. Low cholesterol diets — omit eggs. Use 1 cup liquid egg substitute in step 2.

Brown Bread

Refer to footnotes for special dietary information

INGREDIENTS	WEIGHTS/MEASURES	YIELD ADJUST.	METHOD
All-purpose flour . . . . .1 quart Whole wheat flour. . . . . .1½ quarts Brown sugar . . . . .1 cup Soda .2 tablespoons Nonfat dry milk . . . . .1 cup			1. Place flours, brown sugar, soda and dry milk in mixer bowl and mix at low speed for ½ minute to blend well.
Water. . . . . .1 quart Vinegar . . . . .¼ cup Eggs .1 cup (10 medium) Dark molasses . . . . .2 cups			2. Combine water, vinegar, eggs and molasses and mix until smooth. Add to flour mixture and mix at medium speed until smooth. 3. Pour ¼ of the batter into each of 4 well-greased loaf pans. Bake 40 to 45 minutes or until a cake tester comes out clean from the center. Let set 10 minutes in the pan and then turn out onto a wire rack to cool to room temperature. 4. Cut each loaf into 12 slices about ¾-inch thick.

Cherry Coffee Cake

Refer to footnotes for special dietary information

INGREDIENTS	WEIGHTS/MEASURES	YIELD ADJUST.	METHOD
Margarine ....1 cup (8 ounces) Sugar.....................1⅓ cups Eggs ....1 cup (5-6 medium)			1. Cream margarine and sugar together until light and fluffy. Add eggs and continue to beat at medium speed until well blended.
All-purpose flour ....3 cups Nonfat dry milk ....½ cup Baking powder ....1½ tablespoons Salt ....1 teaspoon			2. Stir flour, dry milk, baking powder and salt together to blend well. Add to creamed mixture and mix at medium speed only until all flour is absorbed.
100% Bran, Bran Buds, All Bran or Fiber One ....1½ cups Water.....................1½ cups			3. Add bran and water to dough. Mix at medium speed only until blended. Spread evenly in well-greased pan.
Canned cherry pie filling......3 cups			4. Using a spoon, place cherry pie filling, using about 2 tablespoonsful at a time, in an even pattern on top of the coffee cake. Using a knife, swirl the pie filling through the dough. 5. Bake 30 to 35 minutes or until the coffee cake is firm in the center. Cut 4 × 6 and serve hot, if possible.

YIELD
24 portions (1 pan)

PORTION SIZE
1 square

PAN SIZE
12 × 18-inch sheet pan

TEMPERATURE
375°F. Oven

NOTE
Other types of pie filling such as apple or apricot may be substituted for the cherry pie filling in step 4.

DIETARY INFORMATION
May be used as written for general, no added salt and bland diets. Low cholesterol diets — omit eggs. Use 1 cup liquid egg substitute in step 1.

YIELD
24 portions (1 pan)

PORTION SIZE
1 square

PAN SIZE
12 × 18-inch sheet pan

TEMPERATURE
350°F. Oven

DIETARY INFORMATION
May be used as written for general, bland and no added salt soft diets. Low cholesterol diets — omit eggs. Use ½ cup liquid egg substitute in step 3.

Cinnamon Raisin Coffee Cake

Refer to footnotes for special dietary information

INGREDIENTS	WEIGHTS/MEASURES	YIELD ADJUST.	METHOD
Sugar	¼ cup		1. Combine sugars, flour, cinnamon and margarine; mix together to form a coarse crumb. Set aside for later use.
Brown sugar	¾ cup		
All-purpose flour	1½ tablespoons		
Cinnamon	1 tablespoon		
Softened margarine	⅓ cup (5⅓ ounces)		
Shortening	1 cup		2. Cream shortening and sugar together at medium speed in mixer bowl until light and fluffy.
Sugar	1½ cups		
Vanilla	2 teaspoons		3. Add vanilla and eggs to creamed mixture and mix at medium speed until creamy.
Eggs	½ cup (2-3 medium)		
All-purpose flour	3 cups		4. Stir flour, baking powder, dry milk and salt together to blend.
Baking powder	1½ tablespoons		
Nonfat dry milk	⅓ cup		
Salt	1 teaspoon		
All Bran, Bran Buds, 100% Bran or Fiber One	1½ cups		5. Add bran, water and raisins along with flour mixture to creamed mixture. Mix at medium speed only until flour is moistened.
Water	1½ cups		6. Spread batter evenly in well-greased pan. Sprinkle topping evenly over batter. Press topping lightly into batter.
Raisins	1 cup		7. Bake 30 to 35 minutes or until cake springs back when touched lightly in the center. Cut 4 × 6 and serve hot, if possible.

Coconut Chocolate Coffee Cake

Refer to footnotes for special dietary information

INGREDIENTS	WEIGHTS/MEASURES	YIELD ADJUST.	METHOD
Flaked coconut . . . . .2 cups Sugar. . . . . .1 cup Softened margarine . . . . .½ cup (8 ounces) Vanilla . . . . .2 teaspoons Chocolate chips . . . . .1 cup (6 ounces)			1. Place coconut, sugar, margarine and vanilla in a small bowl and mix with a spoon to form a coarse crumb. Add chocolate chips and mix lightly. Set aside for use in step 4.
Margarine . . . . .1 cup (8 ounces) Sugar. . . . . .1½ cups Eggs .1 cup (10-12 medium) Vanilla . . . . .2 teaspoons Sour cream . . . . .2 cups			2. Cream margarine and sugar together until light and fluffy. Add eggs, vanilla and sour cream and mix at medium speed until smooth and creamy.
All-purpose flour . . . . .1 quart Soda .2 teaspoons Baking powder . . . . .2 teaspoons Salt . . . . .1 teaspoon			3. Stir flour, soda, baking powder and salt together to blend well. Add to creamy mixture and mix at medium speed until smooth. Spread evenly in well-greased pan. 4. Sprinkle coconut mixture over dough. With a knife or spatula, swirl through the batter to mix the coconut mixture into the batter, being careful not to get the coconut mixture within ½ inch of the edge of the pan. 5. Bake about 20 minutes or until a cake tester comes out clean from the center of the pan and the cake starts to draw away from the sides of the pan. 6. Cut the cake 4 × 6 and serve hot, if possible.

YIELD
24 pieces (1 pan)

PORTION SIZE
1 square

PAN SIZE
12 × 18-inch cake pan

TEMPERATURE
375°F. Oven

VARIATIONS

1. Sour cream coffee cake: Omit ingredients in step 1. Add 1 cup finely chopped pecans and 1 cup washed and drained raisins in step 3.
2. Strawberry sugar coffee cake: Omit ingredients in step 1. Combine ⅓ cup of strawberry-flavored gelatin and 1 cup of sugar. Mix well and substitute for coconut mixture in step 4.
3. Cinnamon-topped coffee cake: Omit ingredients in step 1. Combine 1 cup brown sugar, 2 teaspoons cinnamon and ½ cup softened margarine, mix well and substitute for the coconut mixture in step 4.

DIETARY INFORMATION
May be used as written for general, no added salt and bland diets.

303

YIELD
32 portions (1 pan)

PORTION SIZE
1 square

PAN SIZE
12 × 18-inch cake pan

TEMPERATURE
375°F. Oven

DIETARY INFORMATION
May be used as written for general, no added salt, bland, soft and mechanical soft diets. Diabetic diets — cut the sugar in step 1 to ¼ cup. Each serving, when ¼ cup sugar is used, provides 1 bread and 1 fat exchanges. Low cholesterol diets — omit eggs. Use ¾ cup liquid egg substitute in step 2.

Cornbread

Refer to footnotes for special dietary information

INGREDIENTS	WEIGHTS/MEASURES	YIELD ADJUST.	METHOD
All-purpose flour . . . . .1 quart Cornmeal . . . . .1 quart Nonfat dry milk . . . . .½ cup Sugar. . . . . .½ cup Baking powder . . . . .¼ cup Salt . . . . .2 teaspoons			1. Place flour, cornmeal, dry milk, sugar, baking powder and salt in mixer bowl and mix at low speed for ½ minute to blend well.
Water. . . . . .1 quart Eggs .¾ cup (3-4 medium) Vegetable oil . . . . .1 cup			2. Stir water, eggs and oil together with a fork or whip to blend well; add to flour mixture and mix at medium speed only until all flour is moistened. 3. Spread batter evenly in well-greased pan and bake 30 to 35 minutes or until lightly browned and firm. 4. Cut 4 × 8 and serve hot, if possible.

Dark Bran Muffins

Refer to footnotes for special dietary information

INGREDIENTS WEIGHTS/MEASURES	YIELD ADJUST.	METHOD

All-purpose flour . . . . .1 quart
100% Bran, Bran Buds, All
   Bran or Fiber One . . . . .1½ quarts
Salt . . . . .1 teaspoon
Soda .1½ tablespoons
Sugar. . . . . .1½ cups
Raisins, chopped nuts,
   chopped dates or a
   combination of all of them . .1 quart
		1. Place flour, bran, salt, soda, sugar and raisins or alternates in mixer bowl and mix at low speed for about ½ minute to blend well.

Buttermilk or sour milk . . . . . . .1 quart Molasses . . . . .¾ cup Vegetable oil . . . . .½ cup Eggs .1 cup (5-6 medium)		2. Place buttermilk or sour milk (if sour milk is to be used, pour ¼ cup of white vinegar in a 1-quart measure and fill with whole or 2% milk), molasses, oil and eggs in bowl. Mix to blend well and add all at once to flour mixture. Mix at medium speed only to blend. 3. Fill muffin tins which have been well greased, sprayed with pan spray or lined with paper or foil liners. Bake about 20 minutes or until muffins spring back when touched in the center. Serve hot, if possible.

YIELD
4 dozen muffins

PORTION SIZE
1 muffin

PAN SIZE
Standard muffin tins

TEMPERATURE
400°F. Oven

DIETARY INFORMATION
May be used as written for general, no added salt and bland diets. Diabetic diets — cut the sugar in step 1 to ½ cup. When the sugar is cut, each serving provides 2 bread and 1 fat exchanges.

YIELD
24 servings (1 pan)

PORTION SIZE
1 square

PAN SIZE
12 × 18-inch cake pan

TEMPERATURE
375°F. Oven

DIETARY INFORMATION
May be used as written for general, no added salt, bland and mechanical soft diets. Low cholesterol diets — omit eggs. Use ½ cup liquid egg substitute in step 3.

Golden Bran Coffee Cake

Refer to footnotes for special dietary information

INGREDIENTS	WEIGHTS/MEASURES	YIELD ADJUST.	METHOD
Sugar	⅓ cup		1. Stir sugars and spice together and set aside for use in step 5.
Brown sugar	⅓ cup		
Cinnamon or cardamom	1 teaspoon		
Margarine	1 cup (8 ounces)		2. Cream margarine and sugar together in mixer bowl at medium speed until light and fluffy.
Sugar	1½ cups		
Eggs	½ cup (2-3 medium)		3. Add eggs and vanilla to creamed mixture and mix at medium speed until creamy.
Vanilla	1 tablespoon		
All-purpose flour	1 quart		4. Stir flour, dry milk, baking powder, cinnamon or cardamom together to blend well. Add flour mixture to creamed mixture along with water, bran and salt and mix at medium speed only until all flour is moistened.
Nonfat dry milk	½ cup		
Baking powder	3 tablespoons		
Cinnamon or cardamom	1 teaspoon		
Water at room temperature	2 cups		5. Spread batter evenly in well-greased pan. Sprinkle evenly with sugar mixture and bake about 30 minutes or until lightly browned and the coffee cake starts to pull away from the sides of the pan.
100% Bran, All Bran, Bran Buds or Fiber One	2 cups		
Salt	1 teaspoon		6. Cut 4 × 6 and serve warm, if possible.

Whole Wheat Cinnamon Rolls

Refer to footnotes for special dietary information

YIELD
6 dozen rolls (2 pans)

PORTION SIZE
1 roll

PAN SIZE
12 × 18-inch sheet pans

TEMPERATURE
375°F. Oven

INGREDIENTS	WEIGHTS/MEASURES	YIELD ADJUST.	METHOD
Very hot water . . . . .3½ cups Sugar. . . . . .1 cup Nonfat dry milk . . . . .¾ cup Active dry yeast. . . . . .2 tablespoons			1. Place hot water in mixer bowl; add sugar and dry milk and mix lightly to dissolve sugar; cool to between 110 and 115°F. Add yeast; mix lightly and let set for 5 minutes.
Bread flour . . . . .1½ quarts			2. Add bread flour to liquid and beat at medium speed, using dough hook, for 4 minutes.
Softened margarine . . . . .1 cup (8 ounces) Eggs .1 cup (5-6 medium) Salt . . . . .1 tablespoon Whole wheat flour. . . . . .1½ quarts			3. Add margarine, eggs, salt and whole wheat flour to the batter. Mix at medium speed for 4 minutes.
All-purpose flour . . . . .2 cups Vegetable oil . . . . .2 tablespoons			4. Place flour on working surface. Turn dough out onto flour and knead lightly, using as much of the flour as necessary, to form a smooth resilient dough. Shape dough into a round ball and place in a well-greased bowl. Brush the top of the ball lightly with vegetable oil. Cover with a clean cloth and let stand at room temperature until dough has doubled in volume. 5. Turn dough out onto lightly floured working surface. Knead lightly. Divide dough into 3 equal portions of about 2 pounds, 10 ounces each. Round each portion into a ball. Place balls on a lightly floured working surface, cover with a clean cloth and let the dough rest for 10 minutes.
Softened margarine . . . . .¾ cup (6 ounces) Brown sugar . . . . .2 cups Sugar. . . . . .2 cups Ground cinnamon. . . . . .2 tablespoons			6. Use about ½ of the margarine to heavily grease 2 sheet pans. Mix sugars and cinnamon and sprinkle ¼ of the mixture evenly over the margarine in each pan. 7. Roll each ball of dough out into a 9 × 16-inch rectangle. Spread ⅓ of the remaining margarine evenly over each piece of dough, leaving about ½ inch of the outside free of margarine.

VARIATIONS
1. Whole wheat cinnamon raisin rolls: Sprinkle ½ cup washed and drained raisins on top of the sugar mixture in step 8.
2. Whole wheat pecan rolls: Omit cinnamon in step 6. Sprinkle 1 cup coarsely chopped pecans on the sugar mixture in step 6.

DIETARY INFORMATION
May be used as written for general, bland and no added salt diets. Low cholesterol diets — omit eggs. Use 1 cup liquid egg substitute in step 3.

Continues on next page

Continued from preceding page

INGREDIENTS	WEIGHTS/MEASURES	YIELD ADJUST.	METHOD
			8. Sprinkle 1/3 of the remaining sugar mixture evenly over the margarine on each rectangle. Roll into long rolls and cut each roll into 24 equal slices. 9. Place slices 9 × 4 on top of margarine and sugar in each sheet pan. Cover with a cloth and let rise in a warm place until doubled in volume. 10. Bake 25 to 30 minutes or until golden brown. Turn rolls upside down onto a cooling rack when they are baked. Serve warm, if possible.

Bran Squares for Diabetics

Refer to footnotes for special dietary information

INGREDIENTS	WEIGHTS/MEASURES	YIELD ADJUST.	METHOD

All-purpose flour . . . . .1½ cups
100% Bran, Bran Buds, All
   Bran or Fiber One . . . . .1½ cups
Brown sugar . . . . .¼ cup
Nonfat dry milk . . . . .⅓ cup
Baking powder . . . . .4 teaspoons
Salt . . . . .½ teaspoon
Sugar substitute . . . . .equal to
                ½ cup sugar
			1. Place flour, bran, brown sugar, dry milk, baking powder and salt in mixer bowl. Mix at low speed to blend well.

Water at room temperature. . . .1¼ cups Vegetable oil . . . . .⅓ cup Eggs .½ cup (2-3 medium)			2. Combine water, oil and eggs and mix to blend with a fork. Add to flour and mix at medium speed only until all flour is moistened. 3. Pour batter into well-greased pan and bake 25 to 30 minutes or until firm in the center. 4. Cut 3 × 6 and serve warm, if possible.

YIELD
18 servings (1 pan)

PORTION SIZE
1 square

PAN SIZE
9 × 13-inch cake pan

TEMPERATURE
400°F. Oven

VARIATION
Polka dot bread for diabetics: Add 1 cup washed and drained raisins in step 2. Diabetic exchanges remain the same as for the basic recipe when the bread is cut into 20 portions.

DIETARY INFORMATION
May be used as written for general, no added salt, low fat, bland and mechanical soft diets. Diabetic diets — each serving provides 1 bread and 1 fat exchanges. Low cholesterol diets — omit eggs. Use ½ cup liquid egg substitute in step 2.

Index